Contemporary Diagnosis and Management of

Respiratory Syncytial Virus®

Leonard E. Weisman, MD, Editor

Professor of Pediatrics
Head, Section of Neonatology
Director, Neonatal-Perinatal Medicine
Fellowship, Baylor College of Medicine,
and Chief, Neonatology Service,
Texas Children's Hospital, Houston, Texas

Jessie R. Groothuis, MD, Editor

Medical Director, Anti-Infectives,
Abbott International Division
Abbott Laboratories
Abbott Park, Illinois

D0288758

First Edition
Published by Handbooks in Health Care Co.,
Newtown, Pennsylvania

International Standard Book Number: 1-884065-90-2

Library of Congress Catalog Card Number: 00-09437

Table of Contents

This book has been prepared and is presented as a service to the medical community. The information provided reflects the knowledge, experience, and personal opinions of Leonard E. Weisman, MD, Professor of Pediatrics, Head, Section of Neonatology, Director, Neonatal-Perinatal Medicine Fellowship, Baylor College of Medicine, Houston, Texas, and Jessie R. Groothuis, MD, Medical Director, Anti-Infectives, Abbott International Division, Abbott Laboratories, Abbott Park, Illinois, and of the authors who contributed individual chapters.

This book is not intended to replace or to be used as a substitute for the complete prescribing information prepared by each manufacturer for each drug. Because of possible variations in drug indications, in dosage information, in newly described toxicities, in drug/drug interactions, and in other items of importance, reference to such complete prescribing information is definitely recommended before any of the drugs discussed are used or prescribed.

 *Chapter* **1**

Introduction

S ince its initial isolation in 1956, respiratory syncytial virus (RSV) has become recognized as a
major health problem throughout the world. RSV
is an ubiquitous pathogen that yearly causes seasonal epidemics in all ages. Primary infection usually occurs in
children before 2 years of age, with a peak incidence at 2
to 8 months of age. In older children and adults, RSV generally manifests as a mild upper respiratory tract infection. However, in immunocompromised individuals, those
with underlying cardiopulmonary disorders, preterm infants, and other vulnerable groups, RSV can cause severe
or even fatal bronchiolitis or pneumonia. In the United
States alone, RSV results in the hospitalization of more
than 100,000 infants and children each year, at an estimated annual cost exceeding $500 million.

In recent years, we have witnessed an explosion of new
and exciting information about RSV and its resulting infection. This has led to improved recognition, prevention,
and treatment strategies and has markedly improved outcomes in our most vulnerable populations. Clinicians now
have the ability to help their patients in a meaningful way
and researchers are pushing the frontiers of science forward with advances using the latest molecular techniques.
Clearly, the present is better and the future looks brighter
as we work toward the eradication of this disease.

Although much has been learned about this virus and
the host's response to it, many hurdles still remain before

it can be regarded as a universally preventable disease. This handbook is designed to provide clinicians and researchers with the most current review of RSV and the disease it causes. It includes chapters devoted to the history, properties, animal models, epidemiology, risk factors, clinical characteristics, differential diagnosis, pathology, immune response, laboratory diagnosis, therapy, current prevention strategies, future prevention strategies, and economics of RSV infection.

We are fortunate to have world-renowned experts in this field contribute chapters to this book and we appreciate their efforts to provide this valuable reference to our readers. We hope this text will become a resource for clinicians and researchers in their efforts to provide their patients with the best care now and in the future.

We are pleased to see this handbook on RSV infection come to fruition. We would like to acknowledge several individuals for their technical and administrative assistance, including Marlane Kayfes, Christopher Yeager, Juan Moreno, Carolyn Brewington, Brendie Barrineau, and Diana Wright. We would also like to recognize the support of our families since they, too, have always made an extra effort for those to whom we dedicate this book—our patients.

Leonard E. Weisman, MD
Jessie R. Groothuis, MD

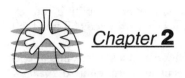

Chapter **2**

Respiratory Syncytial Virus: A Brief History

Val G. Hemming, MD

F. Edward Hébert School of Medicine,
Uniformed Services University of the Health Sciences
Bethesda, Maryland

Scientific progress is not linear. New scientific or medical knowledge often comes in fits and starts, and sometimes arrives in unexpected ways. The history of a ubiquitous human respiratory tract virus, now called respiratory syncytial virus (RSV), is a striking illustration of the unexpected. The first clinical description of RSV illness in young infants was written by John Eberle more than 150 years ago:

"*Congestive Catarrhal Fever*. Infants are liable to a catarrhal affection... the disease commences with cough, and breathing soon becomes laborious and wheezing...The cough is at first dry, attended with a wheezing sound in the chest; but towards the termination of the complaint, it frequently becomes humid and rattling...There is constantly much difficulty breathing, but at times, the oppression becomes so great as to resemble a violent attack of asthma...It is most frequently met in infants under a year old, and I have witnessed several cases during the first month."[1]

This recognizable description of bronchiolitis in infancy suggests that RSV infections have afflicted children for a long time.

In 1941, John Adams described a severe clinical epidemic of respiratory illness in newborns entitled, *Primary virus pneumonitis with cytoplasmic inclusion bodies: study of an epidemic involving 32 infants with 9 deaths*. He wrote:

"The present report deals with a hitherto undescribed form of epidemic pulmonary disease occurring in newborn infants. Its peculiar symptomatology and pathology, as well as its epidemic character, clearly indicate the viral nature of its etiology. Characteristic cytoplasmic inclusion bodies were found in the bronchial epithelium of all fatal cases...The 32 cases reported here occurred in rapid succession during the 3 winter months January, February and March 1937...The characteristic clinical signs of the disease were cough, dyspnea, cyanosis, and low-grade fever...Early in the clinical course fine rales could usually be heard over the chest, indicating involvement of the smaller bronchiolar system...Evidence of dullness indicating consolidation was rarely found. It was practically impossible to determine by physical examination whether or not bronchiolitis or bronchopneumonia was present."[2]

Adams observed and reported on a second epidemic of bronchiolitis and pneumonia, also in Minnesota, in the winter of 1940-1941.[3,4] His laboratory studies, using pathologic materials from some of the deceased infants, effectively ruled out bacteria and rickettsia as causes for the epidemics. In January through March 1961, Adams, then in Los Angeles, observed a third epidemic of bronchiolitis and pneumonia in infants and young children that resembled the two he reported 20 years earlier in Minnesota. By 1961, RSV had been isolated and described. Adams isolated RSV from many of his patients during the 1961 epidemic. Comparing the 3 epidemics, he wrote:

"Unfortunately, proof that this epidemic, most probably related to the RS virus, is identical with the epidemic observed in 1937 will never be established...The epidemic is similar in its epidemiological, clinical, and pathological aspects to an epidemic of pneumonitis in infants characterized by giant cells and cytoplasmic inclusion bodies first reported in 1941."[5]

These observations demonstrate that epidemics of RSV bronchiolitis and pneumonia in North America were not new when the first actual RSV reports were published between 1956 and 1961. Only during this time, however, was RSV actually cultured and described.

The concept of a filterable virus as the cause for tobacco mosaic disease was reported in 1892 by Dimitri Ivanovski. His observations showed that there were pathogenic life forms much smaller than bacteria and fungi. Despite steady progress in virology, by the early 1950s, the viral agent responsible for epidemic bronchiolitis and pneumonia in infants remained unknown.

Several interesting coincidences surround the recovery and characterization of the virus responsible for epidemic bronchiolitis and pneumonia in infants. In 1890, United States Army Surgeon General George Miller Sternberg, an accomplished bacteriologist, appointed Major Walter Reed, a veteran Army physician and surgeon, and later a faculty member of the Army Medical School at Washington, DC, to lead the US Army Commission on Yellow Fever. In 1900, Reed and his colleagues identified the yellow fever virus, the first virus proven to be responsible for a human disease. He reported that yellow fever was a viral zoonosis transferred from monkeys to humans by Aedes mosquitoes. After his untimely death in 1902, Reed became an icon for military and scientific medicine in the 20th century.[6]

Some 55 years later, in October 1955, at the Walter Reed Army Institute of Research (WRAIR) in suburban Washington, DC, several young chimpanzees housed for medical experiments became ill with sneezing and a copious mucopurulent nasal discharge. J.A. Morris, a WRAIR investigator, and his associates recovered a new virus from the monkeys' nasal secretions. They named this new virus *chimpanzee coryza agent* (CCA). They were able to induce the same respiratory illness in nonimmune chimpanzees by intranasal challenge with the new agent.[7] While CCA repli-

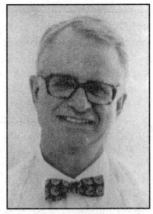

Figure 1: *Robert M. Chanock, MD.*

cated in vitro in human liver epithelial cells, it failed to infect chick embryos or replicate in vivo in other laboratory animals. While these studies were in progress, a WRAIR laboratory worker also developed cold symptoms. Although CCA was not recovered from his throat, he subsequently developed convalescent CCA antibody titers. CCA antibodies were also found in randomly selected sera from patients at the Walter Reed Army Medical Center, suggesting past infection with CCA or a related virus. Interestingly, the respected American virologist Joseph E. Smadel, a colleague of Robert M. Chanock, 'introduced' the Morris CCA report.[8] But it was Chanock who first described and named respiratory syncytial virus (RSV) in infants and young children. Chanock (Figure 1), a pediatrician and virologist, trained in the laboratory of Albert Sabin.

In 1956, Chanock was conducting studies in infants with respiratory tract infections at the Harriet Lane Home in Baltimore, Maryland. He recovered a CCA-like virus from an infant with bronchiolitis and from another infant with pneumonia. Phenotypic and serologic comparisons of these human respiratory viruses with CCA found them to be indistinguishable. Chanock examined convalescent sera from infants with seasonal, and presumed viral, lower respiratory tract infections (LRTIs), and compared the results with age-matched control infants without LRTIs. Many infants and children with LRTIs developed humoral immunity to the CCA-like viruses during the 5 months of observation. The strains of virus from his 2 infants with bronchiolitis and pneumonia replicated in cell culture. The infected cells exhibited a striking cytopathologic effect consisting of multinucleated giant cells circumscribed by large syncytia. Consequently, Chanock proposed respiratory syncytial virus as a more suitable name than CCA.[9,10]

In short order, after the initial CCA/RSV reports, workers in Chicago and Philadelphia confirmed that a CCA-like virus was responsible for epidemic outbreaks of human respiratory illnesses, with a spectrum of severity from mild upper respiratory signs and symptoms to severe and serious LRTIs in patients ranging in age from 1 month to adult. Chanock, at NIH, teamed with Robert H. Parrott (Figure 2) and his colleagues at the Children's Hospital National Medical Center in Washington, DC to conduct extended longitudinal studies on the epidemiology of the now-called RS virus and to characterize the range of clinical manifestations of RSV-induced disease. In 1961, they described the range of clinical manifestations, observed the annual seasonal outbreaks, identified the problem of recurrence of RSV infection in childhood, and began the development of an RSV vaccine.[11,12] In 1958, in consultation with Chanock, Marc Beem et al in Chicago successfully isolated and characterized 41 strains of RSV from 291 patients, exhibiting a spectrum of disease that included mild upper respiratory tract infection, bronchiolitis, pneumonia, and croup.[13]

Numerous reports throughout the 1960s confirmed that RSV was a common cause of seasonal epidemics of mild to serious respiratory infections in infants and children

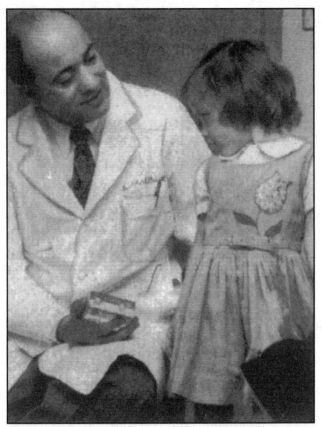

Figure 2: Robert H. Parrott, MD (1923-1999).

throughout the world. In most communities, RSV infections occurred annually, often in widespread winter epidemics, and led to the hospitalization of many infants. Nearly all children studied were found to have been infected with RSV in their first 2 years of life. RSV was also recovered from adults with respiratory infections. It became evident, therefore, that primary RSV infections may not confer solidly protective or durable immunity.

Indeed, in 1960, Johnson and Chanock infected and caused RSV illness in adult volunteers with prechallenge humoral immunity.[14]

The successful development of the Salk polio vaccine and the apparent frequency and morbidity of RSV infections suggested that an RSV vaccine might be similarly developed. Vaccine development for RSV began in the early 1960s; by the mid 1960s, RSV antigen-containing vaccines had undergone animal testing and some limited testing in humans.[15] The Merck Institute for Therapeutic Research developed and tested polyvalent vaccines containing formalin 'killed' RSV mixed with killed parainfluenza and *Mycoplasma pneumoniae* antigens.[16]

Contemporaneously, Chanock et al at NIH developed, and, in partnership with Parrott and associates, began testing a formalin-inactivated RSV vaccine.[17] The NIH-sponsored clinical trials, using a formalin-inactivated, 100-fold concentrated, alum-precipitated RSV vaccine (Lot 100), were conducted in the mid 1960s at 2 sites in Washington, DC, and in military-dependent children at Fitzsimmons Army Hospital and Lowry Air Force Base in Colorado and at Fort Ord Army Hospital in California. About 9 months after completion of the 3-dose immunization schedules in the enrolled infants, epidemics of RSV occurred in the communities where the enrollees lived. Vaccinated infants experienced RSV infections at rates similar to control patients who had received only a formalin-inactivated parainfluenza vaccine. However, 80% of infected vaccinees developed pneumonia or bronchiolitis and required hospitalization, compared to just 5% of the control patients. Two of the vaccine recipients, hospitalized with RSV infection, died in January 1967 at Children's Hospital in Washington. What happened? Why was the vaccine not protective and why was pulmonary disease accentuated in the postvaccinated, RSV-infected children? Though much work has been done over the ensuing 30 years, no fully satisfactory explanation has been found. These unexplained details have loomed over many subsequent efforts to develop safe RSV vaccines to protect infants.

Seeking to explain the enhanced disease in the vaccinated infants, one clinician initially suggested that "the natural RS bronchiolitis that affects young infants who have natural antibody could be described as a variety of Arthus-type reaction in the lung. The virus multiplies in the respiratory tract and produces sufficient antigen to be precipitated in vessels around the bronchioles by circulating maternal antibody. Similarly, multiplication occurs in older children who have been given killed vaccine and is precipitated by an antibody made in response to the vaccine."[18] This unproven hypothesis was assimilated into the medical literature and was taught— almost as dogma— to a generation of medical practitioners. Its acceptance probably hindered the search for better ways to prevent or treat RSV for at least a dozen years.

Subsequent efforts to develop a safe, protective RSV vaccine for infants included preparation of live-attenuated or cold-adapted mutant RSV strains for injection or for intranasal inoculation. Portions of the RSV genome were inserted into other virus vectors, such as vaccinia. Affinity-purified natural or recombinant DNA-derived subunit vaccines were prepared containing surface proteins known to provoke neutralizing antibodies after natural infection. Several complex issues have complicated these efforts. Vaccine safety remains a serious concern because of the failed 1966-1967 killed-RSV vaccine trial. Many infants have passively-acquired maternal circulating RSV antibodies but still become infected. It is well known that many infants with primary RSV infections in the first year of life experience another RSV infection in their second year of life. If natural RSV infection does not provide protective immunity, then any candidate vaccine must enhance immunity well beyond that which results from the natural infection.

Although RSV preferentially replicates in nasal and bronchial epithelial cells, little is known about pathologic changes occurring in the airways of patients with uncomplicated RSV infection, as these are nearly always self-limited. It is probably uncommon for RSV to be carried to organ systems beyond the respiratory tract. Despite this, there is an apparent association of viral respiratory tract infections, especially RSV, with episodes of neonatal apnea and with sudden infant death syndrome (SIDS). Typical is the report by Bruhn et al.[19] In a retrospective review of 274 infants under 6 months of age with culture-proved RSV infection, apnea was observed in 56. Apnea was more likely to occur in prematurely born or term-born infants less than 1 month of age. The occurrence of apnea is unrelated to the severity of the lower respiratory tract symptoms and may, in fact, precede other symptoms. By mechanisms not yet understood, it appears that RSV may play a role in some episodes of SIDS in infants and young children.[20]

The ubiquity and seriousness of RSV infections, and the difficulty in developing an effective vaccine reinforced the requirement to develop in vivo models of RSV infection. The first animal model of RSV infection was the accidental infection of the Walter Reed chimpanzees. Chimpanzees are not available in sufficient numbers for RSV trials and costs prohibit their general use. Morris subsequently attempted to replicate RSV in chicken eggs, mice, guinea pigs, and rabbits. Later, infant ferrets and several primate species other than chimpanzees were also found to be permissive for RSV. An important animal model was reported by Gregory Prince (Figure 3), Robert Chanock, et al in 1978.[21] The cotton rat, a rodent native to North and Central America, has made valuable contributions to our understanding of the pathogenesis of RSV infections. It was critical in the development of RSV immunoprophylaxis and has permitted improved safety testing of RSV vaccines. The model also provided critical in vivo evidence that the hypothesized pulmonary Arthus-type, antigen-antibody reaction played little or no role in RSV bronchiolitis in young infants.[22,23]

At least 3 areas of investigation are prominent in the enormous RSV medical and microbiologic literature. One is the abundant descriptive and microbiologic data on the epidemiology of RSV in human populations; a second is the structural, biochemical, and genetic characterization of the virus; and a third is the expanding list of risk factors responsible for serious RSV disease.

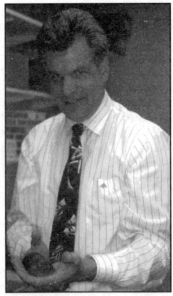

Figure 3: Gregory A. Prince, DDS, PhD, and the cotton rat.

Chanock, Parrott, and colleagues documented the clinical syndromes, seasonality, and epidemiology of RSV in 21,000 infected patients over 13 years in Washington, DC.[24,25] Carl Brandt, the laboratory virologist at Children's Hospital during most of these years, described the difficult logistic, laboratory, and clinical challenges he and his coinvestigators experienced during these protracted studies. They collected, recorded, and collated large amounts of laboratory, clinical, and epidemiologic data before the advent of modern laboratory automation and data management with computers. He recounted: "This was done by writing our data on great big rolls. Dr. Kim's team would keep track of each individual patient, the various isolates, serologic results, and then record it all on large, scrolled wall charts. From these wall charts, we collated data for the various RSV infections and used these as our references."[26] He further reported that Children's now has more than 40 years of RSV data and has documented that a winter RSV epidemic has occurred in Washington, DC every year since 1957.

Caroline Breese Hall's (Figure 4) impressive clinical contributions to the understanding of RSV infections is

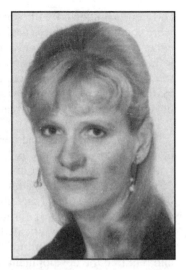

Figure 4: *Caroline Breese Hall, MD.*

another major part of the RSV story. Her work, in collaboration with numerous colleagues, spans more than 25 years. She reported improved methods for RSV isolation and characterization, verified the seasonality of RSV epidemics,[27] quantified the associated hospitalization rates, confirmed much about the clinical syndromes, and broadened understanding of the populations at risk. She documented the serious risks for the newborn and characterized the problems of nosocomial spread of RSV in hospitalized infants and children, as well as quantifying the risks for adults who care for these children. Dr. Hall helped develop approaches to prevent nosocomial spread of RSV in inpatients and identified infection risks for neonates, children with compromised immune systems, and those with congenital heart disease. She verified the problem of reinfection with RSV, and conducted early studies suggesting that ribavirin might be useful in the therapy of children hospitalized with severe RSV LRTIs. Studies were conducted on illness acuity in infants infected with either A or B strains of the virus. In conclusion, there seems to be almost no major research question regarding RSV to which Caroline Hall has not made a contribution. The world's children are beholden to her for her creativity and devotion to the diagnosis, treatment, and prevention of RSV infections.

By 1963, Bloth et al had described the ultrastructure of RSV, showing that it was 120 to 300 nm in diameter with spikes protruding from its envelope.[28] By the late 1970s, investigators had confirmed that the virus contains a single negative-stranded, nonsegmented RNA and fits within the paramyxovirus group. Characterization of RSV antigens was complicated because most RSV proteins prepared in cell culture remained cell-associated and required the development of immunologic reagents to facilitate purification. In 1980, Bernstein and Hruska immunoprecipitated 5 viral proteins using polyclonal RSV antibodies.[29] They and others used immunoprecipitation to characterize the structural and nonstructural proteins of RSV. Cote et al reported the preparation of RSV monoclonal antibodies by 1981, which permitted more accurate functional and structural characterization of RSV proteins.[30] Soon, as many as 9 virus-encoded proteins were detected.[31] Additional reports appeared throughout the 1980s that elucidated much about the virus' genetic and biochemical structure.

Noteworthy in the biochemical and genetic characterization of RSV is the nearly 20 years of study by Gail Wertz and Peter Collins. By 1984, they confirmed 10 viral genes and their polypeptide products, including the critical F and G glycoproteins.[32] Their investigations, and complementary investigations by many others, confirmed that the human antibody response following RSV infection was mainly directed at 3 proteins (30K, 48K, and 72K).[33] The 48K glycoprotein is responsible for cell-to-cell fusion and the formation of syncytia. The large G glycoprotein is responsible for attachment to respiratory epithelial cells.[34]

Modern medicine has created new human populations whose pulmonary or immune systems are compromised. Many premature infants, who were not viable 25 years ago, survive at rates exceeding 90% because of new medical interventions. Many of these infants fare poorly when infected with RSV.[35] Aggressive immune suppression is used widely for organ transplantation and treatment of cancer. Children with chronic pulmonary disorders, such as cystic fibrosis, are living well into adulthood. People are living longer and more are finding nursing home care necessary near the ends of their lives. To no one's surprise, the ubiquitous RSV has become a serious threat to persons in each of these groups.[36] Preventive and treatment strategies must be improved.

The seeming promise of ribavirin has not been borne out and recommendations for its use have been tempered.[37] The development of polyclonal human RSV-immune globulin (RSV-IGIV, RespiGam™) and RSV-specific monoclonal antibodies with neutralizing activity (palivizumab, Synagis™) promised new therapies for RSV infection. However, similar to the ribavirin trials, studies have indicated that antibody therapy was less efficacious than expected. Several large treatment trials yielded results similar to the initial 1987 immunoglobulin treatment trial.[38] Much more positive has been the development of passive immunization for the prevention of RSV with RSV-IGIV and palivizumab.[39,40] Immunoprophylaxis has significantly reduced RSV-related hospitalizations and disease severity in premature infants who received monthly injections during the winter season. Palivizumab is now being used in North America and is licensed throughout the world for the prevention of RSV LRTIs in preterm infants with and without chronic lung disease. Similar preventive strategies are being considered for other high-risk populations.

A number of vaccines are undergoing clinical testing. Antiviral drugs are also being tested. Combined drug therapy trials are under consideration to test whether simultaneously reducing virus replication and the respiratory tract inflammatory response may enhance recovery. Despite 45 years of intensive and fruitful research, RSV's interaction with its host remains enigmatic and poorly understood. The RSV story has many more chapters to be written and will likely provide additional surprises.

References

1.   Eberle J: *A Treatise on the Diseases and Physical Education of Children*. Philadelphia, Lippincott, Grambo and Co, 1850, pp 322-323.

2.   Adams JM: Primary virus pneumonitis with cytoplasmic inclusion bodies. *JAMA* 1941;116:925-933.

3.   Adams JM, Green RG, Evans CA, et al: Primary viral pneumonitis: a comparative study of two epidemics. *J Pediatr* 1942;20:405-420.

4.   Adams JM: A new form of virus pneumonitis occurring epidemically among newborn infants. *Proc Soc Exp Med* 1941;46:114-116.

5.   Adams JM, Imagawa DT, Zike K: Epidemic bronchiolitis and pneumonitis related to respiratory syncytial virus. *JAMA* 1961;176:1037-1039.

6.   Kelly HA: *Walter Reed and Yellow Fever*. New York, McClure, Phillips and Co, 1906, pp 120-123.

7.   Morris JA, Blount RE Jr, Savage RE: Recovery of cytopathogenic agent from chimpanzees with coryza. *Proc Soc Exper Biol Med* 1956;92:544-549.

8.   Crumrine M: Sought copies of the original data from the Morris et al Chimpanzee studies and reported that the documents were probably destroyed when WRAIR moved to its new facilities in 1999. Personal communication.

9.   Chanock R, Rozman B, Myers R: Recovery from infants with respiratory illness of a virus related to chimpanzee coryza agent (CCA): I. Isolation, properties and characterization. *Am J Hyg* 1957;66:281-290.

10.   Chanock R, Finberg L: Recovery from infants with respiratory illness of a virus related to chimpanzee coryza agent (CCA): II. Epidemiologic aspects of infection in infants and young children. *Am J Hyg* 1957;66:291-300.

11.   Chanock RM, Kim HW, Vargosko AJ, et al: Respiratory syncytial virus: I. Virus recovery and other observations during a 1960 outbreak of bronchiolitis, pneumonia, and minor respiratory diseases in children. *JAMA* 1961;176:647-653.

12.   Parrott RH, Vargosko A, Kim HW, et al: Serologic studies over a 34-month period of children with bronchiolitis, pneumonia and minor respiratory diseases. *JAMA* 1961;176:653-657.

13.   Beem M, Wright FH, Hamre D, et al: Association of the chimpanzee coryza agent with acute respiratory disease in children. *N Engl J Med* 1960;263:523-530.

14.   Johnson KM, Chanock RM, Rifkind D, et al: Respiratory syncytial virus: IV. Correlation of virus shedding, serologic response, and illness in adult volunteers. *JAMA* 1961;176:663-667.

15.   Hilleman MR: Respiratory syncytial virus. *Am Rev Respir Dis* 1963;88:181-197.

16.   Potash L, Tytell AA, Sweet BH, et al: Respiratory virus vaccines. I. Respiratory syncytial and parainfluenza virus vaccines. *Am Rev Respir Dis* 1966;93:536-548.

17.   Kapikian AZ, Mitchell RH, Chanock RM, et al: An epidemiologic study of altered clinical reactivity to respiratory syncytial (RS) virus infection in children previously vaccinated with an inactivated RS virus vaccine. *Am J Epidemiol* 1969;89:405-421.

18.   Jeffcoate TN: Vaccine against respiratory syncytial virus. *Lancet* 1969;2:311.

19.   Bruhn FW, Mokrohisky ST, McIntosh K: Apnea associated with respiratory syncytial virus infection in young infants. *J Pediatr* 1977;90:382-386.

20.   Williams AL, Uren EC, Bretherton L: Respiratory viruses and sudden infant death. *Br Med J* 1984;288:1491-1493.

21.   Prince GA, Jenson AB, Horswood RL, et al: The pathogenesis of respiratory syncytial virus infection in cotton rats. *Am J Pathol* 1978;93:771-791.

22.   Prince GA, Hemming VG, Horswood RL, et al: Immunoprophylaxis and immunotherapy of respiratory syncytial virus infection in the cotton rat. *Virus Res* 1985;3:193-206.

23. Prince GA, Jenson AB, Hemming VG, et al: Enhancement of respiratory syncytial virus pulmonary pathology in cotton rats by prior intramuscular inoculation of formalin-inactivated virus. *J Virol* 1986;57:721-728.

24. Kim HW, Arrobio JO, Brandt CD, et al: Epidemiology of respiratory syncytial virus infection in Washington, DC. I. Importance of the virus in different respiratory tract syndromes and temporal distribution of infection. *Am J Epidemiol* 1973;98:216-225.

25. Parrott RH, Kim HW, Arrobio JO, et al: Epidemiology of respiratory syncytial virus infection in Washington, DC. II. Infection and disease with respect to age, immunologic status, race and sex. *Am J Epidemiol* 1973;98:289-300.

26. Brandt CD: Interview with the author, November 22, 1999, Bethesda, MD. The author also sought to interview Robert H. Parrott, MD, but failed when Parrott died 26 December 1999. Robert M. Chanock, MD was unavailable for an interview.

27. Hall CB, Douglas RG Jr: Respiratory syncytial virus and influenza: Practical community surveillance. *Am J Dis Child* 1976;130:615-620.

28. Bloth B, Espmartz A, Norrby E, et al: The ultrastructure of respiratory syncytial virus. *Arch Gesamte Virusforsch* 1963;13:582-586.

29. Bernstein JM, Hruska JF: Respiratory syncytial virus proteins: identification by immunoprecipitation. *J Virol* 1981;38:278-285.

30. Cote PJ Jr, Fernie BF, Ford EC, et al: Monoclonal antibodies to respiratory syncytial virus: detection of virus neutralization and other antigen-antibody systems using infected human and murine cells. *J Virol Methods* 1981;3:137-147.

31. Dubovi EJ: Analysis of proteins synthesized in respiratory syncytial virus-infected cells. *J Virol* 1982;42:372-378.

32. Collins PL, Huang YT, Wertz GW: Identification of a tenth mRNA of respiratory syncytial virus and assignment of polypeptides to the 10 viral genes. *J Virol* 1984;49:572-578.

33. Vainionpaa R, Meurman O, Sarkkinen H: Antibody response to respiratory syncytial virus structural proteins in children with acute respiratory syncytial virus infection. *J Virol* 1985;53:976-979.

34. Levine S, Klaiber-Franco R, Paradiso PR: Demonstration that glycoprotein G is the attachment protein of respiratory syncytial virus. *J Gen Virol* 1987;68:2521-2524.

35. Groothuis JR, Gutierrez KM, Lauer BA: Respiratory syncytial virus infection in children with bronchopulmonary dysplasia. *Pediatrics* 1988;82:199-203.

36. Englund JA, Sullivan CJ, Jordan MC, et al: Respiratory syncytial virus infection in immunocompromised adults. *Ann Intern Med* 1988;109:203-208.

37. Reassessment of the indications for ribavirin therapy in respiratory syncytial virus infections. American Academy of Pediatrics Committee on Infectious Diseases. *Pediatrics* 1996;97:137-140.

38. Hemming VG, Rodriguez W, Kim HW, et al: Intravenous immunoglobulin treatment of respiratory syncytial virus infections in infants and young children. *Antimicrob Agents Chemother* 1987;31:1882-1886.

39. Groothuis JR, Simoes EA, Levin MJ, et al: Prophylactic administration of respiratory syncytial virus immune globulin to high-risk infants and young children. The Respiratory Syncytial Immune Globulin Study Group. *N Engl J Med* 1993;329:1524-1530.

40. Palivizumab, a humanized respiratory syncytial monoclonal antibody, reduces hospitalization from respiratory syncytial virus infection in high-risk infants. The Impact-RSV Study Group. *Pediatrics* 1998;102:531-537.

Chapter 3

Animal Models of RSV Infection

Gregory A. Prince, DDS, PhD

Virion Systems, Inc.,
Rockville, Maryland

"For want of a horse, a battle was lost." This venerable maxim can easily be applied to the subject of animal models of respiratory syncytial virus (RSV) infection: for lack of an animal model during the first RSV vaccine trials, critical safety testing could not be performed before human infants were immunized. As detailed in Chapter 2, those RSV formalin-inactivated vaccine trials had disastrous results, and their repercussions for RSV vaccine development continue more than 3 decades later. The lack of animal models in which researchers could test for unpredictable pulmonary-enhanced results led, at first, to the erroneous conclusion that RSV antibody was harmful.[1] This assertion, which was dogma for more than a decade, could not be successfully refuted until the development of appropriate animal models. Ironically, as a result of the development of reliable animal models, RSV antibody, once considered harmful, is now the only means of RSV prophylaxis.

Chimpanzee

RSV is now recognized as the primary cause of pulmonary disease in infants and children throughout the world, and is a major cause of disease in the elderly and in several high-risk adult subpopulations. But initial isolation of RSV did not occur in humans. More than 4 decades ago,[2] an epizootic of upper respiratory tract disease in a colony of chimpanzees yielded a Chimpanzee Coryza Agent virus. A year later, this virus was also recognized as a human pathogen and was renamed respiratory syncytial virus (RSV).

Although RSV-related viruses have also been isolated from cattle,[3] sheep,[4] and goats,[5] the chimpanzee remains the only known animal host of human RSV. While this would seem to make the chimpanzee the best animal model of RSV, 2 factors limit its utility. The first is economic. Although bred in captivity, chimpanzees are limited in availability and are extremely expensive, both to purchase and to care for. Terminal experimentation generally is not permitted, and the cost of life-long maintenance, and the logistics of reselling or transferring animals to other facilities can be prohibitive. As a result, only 1 laboratory in the world has reported RSV experimentation in chimpanzees.[6]

The second factor is scientific. The scarcity of animals necessitates 4 or fewer animals per experimental group, and the occasional use of historical rather than concurrent control animals. Studies have been limited to nasal and tracheal lavage specimens,[7] despite the fact that serious RSV disease in humans is pulmonary, and work in rodent models has demonstrated that the upper and lower respiratory tissue responses to RSV infection differ markedly.[8] Perhaps the greatest concern is the apparent inadequacy of the chimpanzee as an attenuation marker for candidate live-virus vaccines.[9]

In the face of these limiting factors, it is unlikely that chimpanzees will be widely used to shed additional light on important questions of RSV pathogenesis and immunology.

Other Primates

Underlying the use of primates in studying human disease are the implicit assumptions that their closer phylogenetic relationship to humans makes them better biologic models, and that use of primates rather than rodents in preclinical studies is preferred by regulatory agencies, such as the US Food and Drug Administration (FDA). Over the past 2 decades, RSV infection was reported in African green, bonnet, cebus, owl, rhesus, and squirrel monkeys, and in baboons.[6,10-14] Promising results were obtained with some of these species, particularly in the area of vaccine-enhanced RSV disease, but their use is limited by expense, scarcity, lack of inbreeding, and lack of host-specific reagents.

Although monkeys are closer relatives of humans than any of the rodents, no primate model has yet proven to be of greater, or even equal, value to rodent models in determining optimal prevention and treatment modalities, and in understanding the immunology of human RSV disease. Indeed, none of the 3 FDA-approved anti-RSV drugs—ribavirin (Virazole®), RSV-IGIV (RespiGam™), or palivizumab (Synagis™)—underwent primate testing before clinical trials.

Cotton Rat

The first successful small-animal model of RSV was described by Dreizin et al in 1971.[15] Using cotton rats exported to the Soviet Union many years earlier (the cotton rat is a New World rodent), Soviet scientists correctly, though briefly, described the basic pathogenesis of RSV infection. For unknown reasons, this group did not publish further studies using cotton rats. The relative inaccessibility of the paper (published in Russian with a brief English abstract) limited its impact for several years. Its eventual translation into English, coupled with the availability of cotton rats from the Veterinary Resources Branch of the National Institutes of Health, led to confirmation and amplification of Dreizin's work.[16]

When the cotton rat model was being developed, conventional wisdom in the aftermath of the failed vaccine trials held that RSV serum antibody was a cause, rather than a prevention, of enhanced pulmonary disease.[1] Experiments in the cotton rat that challenged this convention used the technique of parabiosis, where 2 animals are linked surgically in a way that they share circulating blood. When an immune animal was linked to a nonimmune animal, complete resistance to pulmonary RSV infection was conferred.[8] Subsequent blood fractionation protocols showed that the antiviral factor was serum immunoglobulin G (IgG).[17]

The cotton rat not only refuted the assertion that serum antibody was harmful, but also served as the model leading to clinical testing of antibody prophylaxis. Protective levels required in cotton rats[18] were higher than could be obtained by simply using generic, plasma-derived human IgG.[19] Therefore, an alternative approach involving the screening of plasma donors and selection only of those with high RSV-neutralizing antibody titers was initiated.[20] Protective RSV-neutralizing antibody titers first found in cotton rats,[21] were subsequently used as targets for successful clinical trials with RSV-hyperimmune polyclonal immunoglobulin,[22,23] leading to FDA approval for RespiGam™ for the prevention of RSV pulmonary disease in high-risk preterm infants with and without chronic lung disease.

Plasma-derived polyclonal IgG, even from donors with high RSV titers, must be given intravenously in large volume, because of the small percentage of the total antibody repertoire specific for RSV. Therefore, a second-generation approach to passive prophylaxis was initiated using a monoclonal antibody (MAb). A 'humanized' version of a mouse MAb against the fusion protein of the virus was highly effective in preventing RSV lower respiratory tract infection in cotton rats.[24] Dosage for subsequent clinical trials was based on data from cotton rats, and successful clinical trials[25] led to FDA approval for the humanized monoclonal antibody Synagis™, the only MAb yet to prevent any kind of infectious disease in controlled clinical trials. Interestingly, FDA approval of both prophylactic drugs was based on preclinical data generated solely in cotton rats, with no primate intermediates.

The use of immunoglobulin as a therapeutic agent was also suggested by cotton rat experiments, which demonstrated that RSV titers in previously infected animals could be reduced below detectable levels within hours of parenteral or topical administration of IgG.[17,26] However, subsequent experiments showed that reduced viral titers alone did not correlate with short-term reversal of lung histopathology. Recent clinical trials of Synagis™ as a therapeutic agent confirmed the observation made in cotton rats, as viral titers in tracheal aspirates of intubated infants were reduced without concomitant improvement in clinical outcome.[27] Disappointing results with Virazole®, the only FDA-approved drug for treating RSV infection,[28] also support a growing awareness that RSV therapy must address more than a reduction in viral load. Recent cotton rat trials suggest that a more successful treatment approach to severe RSV disease should combine an antiviral agent (such as immunoglobulin) with an anti-inflammatory agent.[29,30]

An additional area of cotton rat research has been the testing of candidate RSV vaccines. Several companies conducted efficacy and/or safety tests, including Centre d'Immunologie Pierre Fabre,[31] Pasteur Merieux Connaught,[32] SmithKline Beecham Biologicals,[33] Upjohn,[34] and Wyeth-Lederle Vaccines and Pediatrics.[35]

Mouse

Use of the mouse as a model for RSV was delayed for nearly 2 decades by a report that 4 inbred strains of mice did not develop complement-fixing antibodies after intranasal RSV inoculation.[36] Although the investigators did not indicate that there had been an attempt to isolate infectious virus from mouse lungs, the assumption was that the mouse was not permissive for RSV. A later report described 20 inbred strains that were all permissive for RSV infection,[37] albeit over a range of 2 orders of magnitude, from least (CBA/CaHN) to most permissive (DBA/2N). Since that report, the mouse has become the most widely used animal model of RSV infection. The mouse has several advantages over all other laboratory animals: availability of a vast array of inbred strains (including congenic, transgenic, and knockout); an unparalleled armamentarium of specific reagents for detection and quantitation of cells, cytokines, chemokines, immunoglobulins, and many other host molecules; and low purchase and maintenance costs. The immune system of the mouse has been more thoroughly studied than that of any other laboratory animal, providing an unmatched foundation for studies of RSV-specific immune responses.

Important aspects of immunity to RSV being studied in mice[38-41] include: viral gene products that elicit various aspects of the immune response; the cellular and humoral effectors of immunity; and the role of bone marrow-derived cells (particularly the eosinophil) in primary and secondary infection.

Of more immediate relevance to clinical medicine have been studies of the efficacy and safety of candidate RSV vaccines. Much of the preclinical work on live-attenuated vaccines, the candidate RSV vaccines that are the most advanced through clinical trials, has been done in mice.[42,43]

Equally important to the testing of candidate vaccines are studies of the mechanisms by which the formalin-inactivated vaccine of the 1960s caused enhanced disease. Although a model of vaccine-enhanced disease was first described in the cotton rat,[44] its lack of reagents has resulted in the use of mice in nearly all subsequent studies.[45-47] The definition of histologic, cytokine, and chemokine profiles in animals undergoing primary RSV infection, secondary infection, and challenge following immunization with formalin-inactivated RSV (FI-RSV) will be invaluable in assessing the likely safety of candidate RSV vaccines.

Rat

The rat (*Rattus norvegicus*) was recently used to assess the potential long-term impact of RSV on recurrent wheezing and reactive airway disease. Piedimonte et al demonstrated that Synagis™ inhibits neurogenic inflammation in RSV-infected rats. They hypothesize that by limiting the severity of acute airway inflammation, such prophylaxis may protect against later lower respiratory tract illness.[48]

Cow

Bovine RSV (BRSV), which is related to human RSV, was first identified in cattle 13 years after discovery of human RSV.[3] Subsequent studies showed it to be ubiquitous in cattle herds worldwide, and as important a pathogen in cattle as RSV is in humans.[49] Although logistic hurdles of size, cost, and relative paucity of reagents limit the utility of the bovine model, it is the only defined experimental system in which an RSV virus is being studied in its natural host. To date, the most important contribution of the bovine RSV model is the demonstration that enhanced pulmonary disease similar to that caused by FI-RSV occurs when cattle immunized with FI-BRSV are challenged with live BRSV.[50-52]

Guinea Pig

Although less frequently used than the other RSV models, guinea pigs have the advantage of well-studied airway physiology, particularly as it relates to reactive airway disease. The demonstration of heightened responsiveness to acetylcholine following RSV infection of guinea pigs[53] is an intriguing discovery that may eventually shed light on the ongoing debate over the role of RSV in asthma.[54]

Ferret

Although not used for RSV research in recent years, ferrets are unique among animal models in demonstrating age-dependent and organ-dependent susceptibility to infection. While nasal tissues are susceptible to infection at any age,[55] permissiveness to pulmonary infection is short-lived, diminishing rapidly to the point of complete refraction by 1 month of age. Similar age dependence was reported in organ cultures of ferrets of various ages.[56] It is known that the severity of RSV pulmonary disease in human infants is inversely related to age,[57] and it is possible that the ferret holds some clues to the reasons for this phenomenon.

Summary

The development and use of animal models has been essential in increasing our understanding of RSV disease, and in devising safe and effective strategies for its prevention and treatment. RSV disease in humans is multifaceted, with different risks and disease manifestations in different ages and populations. No single animal model can address all facets of human RSV disease, and each of the models described has certain advantages. It is likely that all of these models will continue to add to our knowledge of this important human pathogen, and the challenge for the scientist will be in determining the best model for the question at hand.

References

1.   Chanock RM, Kapikian AZ, Mills J, et al: Influence of immunological factors in respiratory syncytial virus disease. *Arch Environ Health* 1970;21:347-355.

2.   Morris JA, Blount RE, Savage RE: Recovery of cytopathogenic agent from chimpanzees with coryza. *Proc Soc Exp Biol Med* 1956;92:544-549.

3.   Paccaud MF, Jacquier CL: A respiratory syncytial virus of bovine origin. *Arch Gesamte Virusforsch* 1970;30:327-342.

4.   Trudel M, Nadon F, Simard C, et al: Comparison of caprine, human, and bovine strains of respiratory syncytial virus. *Arch Virol* 1989;107:141-149.

5.   Lehmkuhl HD, Smith MH, Cutlip RC: Morphogenesis and structure of caprine respiratory syncytial virus. *Arch Virol* 1980;65:269-276.

6.   Belshe RB, Richardson LS, London WT, et al: Experimental respiratory syncytial virus infection of four species of primates. *J Med Virol* 1977;1:157-162.

7.   Whitehead SS, Bukreyev A, Teng MN, et al: Recombinant respiratory syncytial virus bearing a deletion of either the NS2 or SH gene is attenuated in chimpanzees. *J Virol* 1999;73:3438-3442.

8.   Prince GA, Horswood RL, Camargo E, et al: Mechanisms of immunity to respiratory syncytial virus in cotton rats. *Infect Immun* 1983;42:81-87.

9.   Crowe JE Jr, Randolph V, Murphy BR: The live attenuated subgroup B respiratory syncytial virus vaccine candidate RSV 2B33F is attenuated and immunogenic in chimpanzees, but exhibits partial loss of the ts phenotype following replication in vivo. *Virus Res* 1999;59:13-22.

10.   Kakuk TJ, Soike K, Brideau RJ, et al: A human respiratory syncytial virus (RSV) primate model of enhanced pulmonary pathology induced with a formalin-inactivated RSV vaccine but not a recombinant FG subunit vaccine. *J Infect Dis* 1993;167:553-561.

11.   Babu PG, Selvan A, Christuraj S, et al: A primate model of respiratory syncytial virus infection. *Indian J Exp Biol* 1998;36:758-762.

12.   Richardson LS, Belshe RB, Sly DL, et al: Experimental respiratory syncytial virus pneumonia in cebus monkeys. *J Med Virol* 1978;2:45-59.

13.   Richardson LS, Belshe RB, London WT, et al: Evaluation of five temperature-sensitive mutants of respiratory syncytial virus in primates: I. Viral shedding, immunologic response, and associated illness. *J Med Virol* 1978;3:91-100.

14.   Hildreth SW, Baggs RB, Eichberg JW, et al: A parenterally administered subunit RSV vaccine: safety studies in animals and adult humans. *Pediatr Res* 1989;25:180A.

15.   Dreizin RS, Vyshnevetskaya LO, Bagdamian EE, et al: Experimental RS virus infection in cotton rats. A viral and immunofluorescent study [in Russian]. *Vopr Virusol* 1971;16:670-676.

16.   Prince GA, Jenson AB, Horswood RL, et al: The pathogenesis of respiratory syncytial virus infection in cotton rats. *Am J Pathol* 1978;93:771-791.

17.   Prince GA, Hemming VG, Horswood RL, et al: Immunoprophylaxis and immunotherapy of respiratory syncytial virus infection in the cotton rat. *Virus Res* 1985;3:193-206.

18.   Prince GA, Horswood RL, Chanock RM: Quantitative aspects of passive immunity to respiratory syncytial virus infection in infant cotton rats. *J Virol* 1985;55:517-520.

19.   Meissner HC, Fulton DR, Groothuis JR, et al: Controlled trial to evaluate protection of high-risk infants against respiratory syncytial virus disease by using standard intravenous immune globulin. *Antimicrob Agents Chemother* 1993;37:1655-1658.

20.   Siber GR, Leszczynski J, Pena-Cruz V, et al: Protective activity of a human respiratory syncytial virus immune globulin prepared from donors screened by microneutralization assay. *J Infect Dis* 1992;165:456-463.

21.   Siber GR, Leombruno D, Leszczynski J, et al: Comparison of antibody concentrations and protective activity of respiratory syncytial virus immune globulin and conventional immune globulin. *J Infect Dis* 1994;169:1368-1373.

22.   Groothuis JR, Simoes EA, Levin MJ, et al: Prophylactic administration of respiratory syncytial virus immune globulin to high-risk infants and young children. The Respiratory Syncytial Virus Immune Globulin Study Group. *N Engl J Med* 1993;329:1524-1530.

23.   Reduction of respiratory syncytial virus hospitalization among premature infants and infants with bronchopulmonary dysplasia using respiratory syncytial virus immune globulin prophylaxis. The PREVENT Study Group. *Pediatrics* 1997;99:93-99.

24.   Johnson S, Oliver C, Prince GA, et al: Development of a humanized monoclonal antibody (MEDI-493) with potent in vitro and in vivo activity against respiratory syncytial virus. *J Infect Dis* 1997;176:1215-1224.

25.   Palivizumab, a humanized respiratory syncytial virus monoclonal antibody, reduces hospitalization from respiratory syncytial virus infection in high-risk infants. IMpact-RSV Study Group. *Pediatrics* 1998;102:531-537.

26.   Prince GA, Hemming VG, Horswood RL, et al: Effectiveness of topically administered neutralizing antibodies in experimental immunotherapy of respiratory syncytial virus infection in cotton rats. *J Virol* 1987;61:1851-1854.

27. Malley R, DeVincenzo J, Ramilo O, et al: Reduction of respiratory syncytial virus (RSV) in tracheal aspirates in intubated infants by use of humanized monoclonal antibody to RSV F protein. *J Infect Dis* 1998;178:1555-1561.

28. Ohmit SE, Moler FW, Monto AS, et al: Ribavirin utilization and clinical effectiveness in children hospitalized with respiratory syncytial virus infection. *J Clin Epidemiol* 1996;49:963-967.

29. Prince GA, Porter DD: Treatment of parainfluenza virus type 3 bronchiolitis and pneumonia in a cotton rat model using topical antibody and glucocorticosteroid. *J Infect Dis* 1996;173:598-608.

30. Prince GA: Respiratory syncytial virus antiviral agents. *Exp Opin Ther Patents* 1999;9:753-762.

31. Power UF, Plotnicky-Gilquin H, Huss T, et al: Induction of protective immunity in rodents by vaccination with a prokaryotically expressed recombinant fusion protein containing a respiratory syncytial virus G protein fragment. *Virology* 1997;230:155-166.

32. Du RP, Jackson GE, Wyde PR, et al: A prototype recombinant vaccine against respiratory syncytial virus and parainfluenza virus type 3. *BioTechnology (NY)* 1994;12:813-818.

33. Prieels J-P: Progress towards the development of RSV vaccine at SmithKline Beecham. Oral presentation, *RSV After 40 Years: An Anniversary Symposium.* Kiawah Island Resort, South Carolina, November 9-12, 1996.

34. Wathen MW, Brideau RJ, Thomsen DR: Immunization of cotton rats with the human respiratory syncytial virus F glycoprotein produced using a baculovirus vector. *J Infect Dis* 1989;159:255-264.

35. Randolph VB, Kandis M, Stemler-Higgins P, et al: Attenuated temperature-sensitive respiratory syncytial virus mutants generated by cold adaptation. *Virus Res* 1994;33:241-259.

36. Coates HV, Chanock RM: Experimental infection with respiratory syncytial virus in several species of animals. *Am J Hyg* 1962;76:302-312.

37. Prince GA, Horswood RL, Berndt JA, et al: Respiratory syncytial virus infection in inbred mice. *Infect Immun* 1979;26:764-766.

38. Openshaw PJ: Immunity and immunopathology to respiratory syncytial virus. The mouse model. *Am J Respir Crit Care Med* 1995;152:S59-S62.

39. Hussell T, Openshaw PJ: Immunological determinants of disease caused by respiratory syncytial virus. *Trends Microbiol* 1996;4:299-300.

40. Graham BS: Immunological determinants of disease caused by respiratory syncytial virus. *Trends Microbiol* 1996;4:290-293.

41. Domachowske JB, Rosenberg HF: Respiratory syncytial virus infection: immune response, immunopathogenesis, and treatment. *Clin Microbiol Rev* 1999;12:298-309.

42. Whitehead SS, Firestone CY, Karron RA, et al: Addition of a missense mutation present in the L gene of respiratory syncytial virus (RSV) cpts530/1030 to RSV vaccine candidate cpts248/404 increases its attenuation and temperature sensitivity. *J Virol* 1999; 73:871-877.

43. Bukreyev A, Whitehead SS, Bukreyeva N, et al: Interferon gamma expressed by a recombinant respiratory syncytial virus attenuates virus replication in mice without compromising immunogenicity. *Proc Nat Acad Sci USA* 1999;96:2367-2372.

44. Prince GA, Jenson AB, Hemming VG, et al: Enhancement of respiratory syncytial virus pulmonary pathology in cotton rats by intramuscular inoculation of formalin-inactivated virus. *J Virol* 1986;57:721-728.

45. Tang YW, Neuzil KM, Fischer JE, et al: Determinants and kinetics of cytokine expression patterns in lungs of vaccinated mice challenged with respiratory syncytial virus. *Vaccine* 1997;15:597-602.

46. Tripp RA, Anderson LJ: Cytotoxic T-lymphocyte precursor frequencies in BALB/c mice after acute respiratory syncytial virus (RSV) infection or immunization with a formalin-inactivated RSV vaccine. *J Virol* 1998;72:8971-8975.

47. Waris ME, Tsou C, Erdman DD, et al: Respiratory syncytial virus infection in BALB/c mice previously immunized with formalin-inactivated virus induces enhanced pulmonary inflammatory response with a predominant Th2-like cytokine pattern. *J Virol* 1996;70:2852-2860.

48. Piedimonte G, King KA, Holmgren NL, et al: A humanized monoclonal antibody against respiratory syncytial virus (palivizumab) inhibits RSV-induced neurogenic-mediated inflammation in rat airways. *Pediatr Res* 2000;47:351-356.

49. Van der Poel WH, Brand A, Kramps JA, et al: Respiratory syncytial virus infections in human beings and in cattle. *J Infect* 1994;29:215-228.

50. Gershwin LJ, Schelegle ES, Gunther RA, et al: A bovine model of vaccine enhanced respiratory syncytial virus pathophysiology. *Vaccine* 1998;16:1225-1236.

51. West K, Petrie L, Haines DM, et al: The effect of formalin-inactivated vaccine on respiratory disease associated with bovine respiratory syncytial virus infection in calves. *Vaccine* 1990;17:809-820.

52. Woolums AR, Singer RS, Boyle GA, et al: Interferon gamma production during bovine respiratory syncytial virus (BRSV) infection is diminished in calves vaccinated with formalin-inactivated BRSV. *Vaccine* 1999;17:1293-1297.

53. Robinson PJ, Hegele RG, Schellenberg RR: Allergic sensitization increases airway reactivity in guinea pigs with respiratory syncytial virus bronchiolitis. *J Aller Clin Immunol* 1997;100:492-498.

54. Johnston SL: Viruses and asthma. *Allergy* 1998;53:922-932.

55. Prince GA, Porter DD: The pathogenesis of respiratory syncytial virus infection in infant ferrets. *Am J Pathol* 1976;82:339-352.

56. Porter DD, Muck KB, Prince GA: The age dependence of respiratory syncytial virus growth in ferret lung can be shown in organ and monolayer cultures. *Clin Immunol Immunopathol* 1980;15:415-423.

57. Henderson FW, Collier AM, Clyde WA, et al: Respiratory syncytial virus infections, reinfections and immunity. *N Engl J Med* 1979;300:530-534.

Chapter 4

Epidemiology and Risk Factors

Penelope H. Dennehy, MD

Professor of Pediatrics,
Brown University School of Medicine,
Associate Director,
Division of Pediatric Infectious Diseases,
Hasbro Children's Hospital, Providence, Rhode Island

Respiratory syncytial virus (RSV) is the most significant cause of acute respiratory tract infections in infants and young children throughout the world. The World Health Organization (WHO) estimates that one third of the 12.2 million annual deaths in children under 5 years are the result of acute infections of the respiratory tract, with RSV, *Streptococcus pneumoniae*, and *Haemophilus influenzae* as the predominant pathogens.[1] In the United States alone, approximately 91,000 infants are hospitalized with RSV infections every year, at an estimated annual cost of $300 million.[2] The burden of RSV infections is even greater than the cost of hospitalization alone if we consider outpatient visits for children and adults, RSV morbidity in patients with underlying conditions, and the impact of widespread morbidity associated with RSV infections in the elderly.

Epidemiology

Geographic and seasonal patterns. Serologic surveys indicate that RSV is present in all geographic and climatic

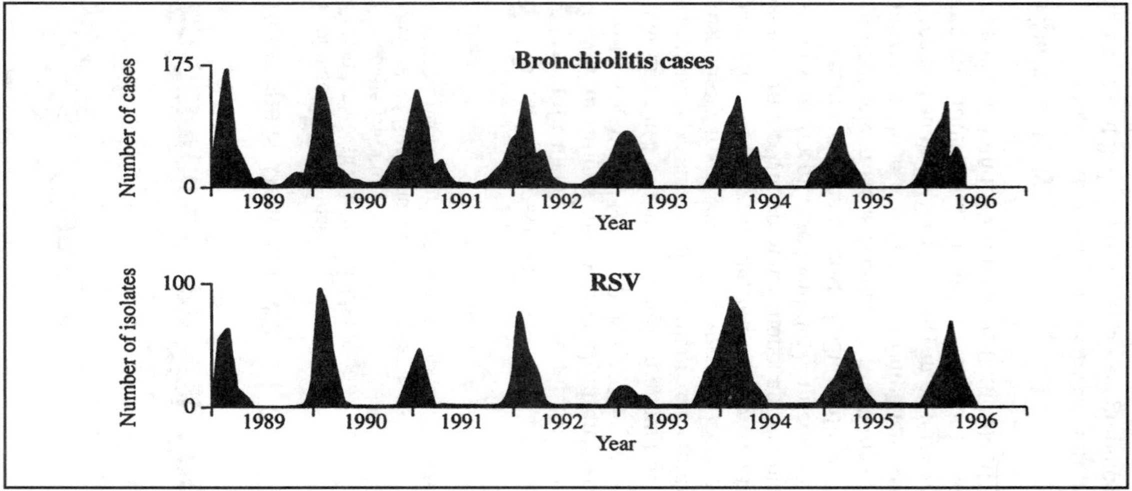

Figure 1: Patterns of reported cases of bronchiolitis in relation to activity of RSV in Monroe County, New York. Data were obtained from a weekly community surveillance program for infectious diseases. Reproduced with permission from: Hall CB: Respiratory syncytial virus: a continuing culprit and conundrum. J Pediatr 1999;135:2-7. Copyright 1999, Mosby Inc.

regions. Clinical manifestations of RSV disease are similar throughout the world,[3-9] but the virus preferentially causes most severe disease in the very young.

RSV causes predictable, widespread outbreaks of illness each year. In temperate climates, RSV infections peak during winter months. Compared with influenza, RSV outbreaks are more gradual in onset and decline. In most areas of the United States, annual outbreaks occur between November and April, occasionally lasting as late as May or June. The highest incidence of disease is in December, January, and February.[10-12] In the southeastern United States, continuous nonseasonal epidemics of RSV infection have been observed.[13] The duration of the outbreaks may vary, but averages 22 weeks.[14] RSV outbreaks occur most frequently in the cold season in areas with Mediterranean climates, and in the wet season in tropical countries with high seasonal rainfall.[9,15] The seasonal patterns on Pacific islands and in areas of the inner tropics with high rainfall levels year-round are less clear.[6]

In the United States, RSV outbreaks in the community are associated with increases in hospital admissions of young children for acute lower respiratory tract disease.[10,16,17] A rise in the number of cases of bronchiolitis or pneumonia in young children seen in pediatric offices and other outpatient settings is also predictive of RSV's arrival in the community (Figure 1).[18] When it is circulating, RSV is usually the dominant respiratory virus in the community.[4] Outbreaks of influenza A may overlap with RSV outbreaks, but the peaks of the epidemics do not commonly coincide.[19]

Strain Variation

The severity of RSV outbreaks varies from year to year,[20] perhaps in part because of a variation in circulating strains. RSV has 2 major antigenic groups, A and B, with additional antigenic variability occurring within each group. The most extensive antigenic and genetic diversity occurs on the G protein on the surface of the virus, which is the attachment glycoprotein.[21] During individual epidemic periods, viruses of both antigenic groups sometimes cocirculate, or viruses of 1 group may predominate. The proportion of each group varies seasonally and geographically, as does the predominance of the A and B strains.[20,22-29] Within each RSV strain, 1 or 2 distinct subgroups predominate in a single year in a given location.[30] Studies of isolates in the United States and the United Kingdom suggest that group A strains predominate in most outbreaks.[20,25,31] Data collected over a 15-year period in Rochester, NY, show a pattern of 1- to 2-year cycles where group A strains predominate, followed by a year in which at least half of the strains are group B. Group A strains predominated in 9 of the 15 years studied, while group B strains predominated in only 2 years a decade apart.[20] In Cannes, France, however, group B strains predominated in 4 of 8 years and accounted for 64% of the total isolates.[32] Over 2 seasons, the strains from 14 cities across the United States varied greatly, suggesting the influence of local, rather than national, factors.[23] Several small studies suggest that homotypic immunity plays a role in the variation of viral strains.[33-35] Thus, the antigenic differences occurring among these viruses may contribute to RSV's ability to establish reinfections throughout life.

The relationship between the circulating strain and the size of the RSV outbreak is not consistent[20]; however, the strain may be associated with clinical severity. In several, although not all, of the studies exploring the association of severity with strain, evidence suggests that group A strains are associated with greater clinical severity.[20,31,36,37]

Acquisition of Infection According to Age

At least 50% of children in the United States contract RSV infection during the first RSV epidemic they encounter, and almost all children are infected by 2 years of age.[5,38] Infection rates peak in infants aged 6 weeks to 6 months, with the highest rates occurring in children under 3 months of age.

The age of the RSV-infected child influences the incidence and type of RSV disease. Lower respiratory tract disease, such as bronchiolitis and pneumonia, is almost always seen in children younger than 3 years, but is relatively uncommon during the first 3 to 4 weeks of life. With increasing age comes a decreasing risk of primary disease and pulmonary involvement. Reinfections are frequent in both older children and adults, most often taking the form of an upper respiratory infection (URI), tracheobronchitis, or reactive airway disease. In the Houston family studies, lower respiratory tract disease occurred in 33% of the children who had RSV infections in the first year of life, and 16% to 23% of the infections in the subsequent 3 years (Table 1).[5]

Incidence and Prevalence

RSV is implicated as the major cause of inpatient and outpatient pneumonia and bronchiolitis in infancy and early childhood in the United States. RSV infection in the young infant produces the greatest morbidity. Forty percent to 90% of bronchiolitis cases are associated with RSV, and during the peak RSV season, 80% or more are RSV-related.[10,16,39,40] RSV accounts for approximately 50% of all pneumonia in infancy,[41] and has been associated with 10% to 30% of pediatric bronchitis.[10] In contrast, fewer than 10% of croup cases are RSV-related.[10,42] RSV is rarely isolated from patients without respiratory disease.[10]

Hospitalization rates for RSV infection are highest in infants between 2 and 6 months of age, with a mean age of approximately 3 months. In Washington, DC, approximately 40% of primary infections involved the lower respiratory tract, and of every 100 primary RSV infections, 1 resulted in a hospital admission for bronchiolitis. RSV-infected children between 2 and 6 months of age com-

Table 1: Frequency of RSV Infection Among Children Studied From Birth*

Age (months)	No. Child-Years of Observation	No. of Primary Infections
0-12	125	85
13-24	92	33
25-36	65	1
37-48	39	0
49-60	24	0
Total	345	119

*Houston Family Study, 1975 through 1980.

Modified with permission from Glezen WP, Taber LH, Frank AL, et al: Risk of primary infection and reinfection with respiratory syncytial virus. *Am J Dis Child* 1986;140:543-546. Copyright 1986, American Medical Association.

prised 75% of the hospitalizations for bronchiolitis and 45% for pneumonia,[8] indicating that the risk of hospitalization for an infant infected with RSV during the first 12 months of life was 1.6%.

Hospitalization rates for RSV infection in the United States vary according to geographic, socioeconomic, and other factors, ranging from approximately 0.1% to 1% of infected infants.[10,40,43-49] A recent analysis of US national hospital discharge survey data from 1980 through 1996 reassessed the estimates of current hospitalizations associated with RSV infection in children younger than 5 years. Fifty-seven percent of the children hospitalized with RSV infection were younger than 6 months, and 81% were younger than 1 year. Among children younger

No. of Reinfections	% of Cohort Infected	% of Cohort With Lower Respiratory Disease
1	68.8	22.4
43	82.6	13.0
29	46.2	10.8
13	33.3	7.7
12	50.0	0
98	62.9	14.5

than 1 year, annual bronchiolitis hospitalization rates increased 2.4-fold, from 12.9 per 1,000 in 1980 to 31.2 per 1,000 in 1996. From 1988 to 1996, infant hospitalization rates for bronchiolitis increased significantly, while those for lower respiratory tract diseases, excluding bronchiolitis, did not vary significantly. The proportion of hospitalizations for lower respiratory tract illnesses among children younger than 1 year associated with bronchiolitis increased from 22.2% in 1980 to 47.4% in 1996; among total hospitalizations, this proportion increased from 5.4% to 16.4%. Averaging bronchiolitis hospitalizations during 1994 to 1996 (assuming that RSV was the etiologic agent in 50% to 80% of November through April hospitalizations), an estimated 51,240 to

81,985 annual bronchiolitis hospitalizations among children younger than 1 year were related to RSV infection.[50] Mortality associated with primary RSV infection in otherwise healthy children is estimated to be 0.005% to 0.02%,[51] and is approximately 1% to 3%[52] among hospitalized children.

RSV infection during the first 4 weeks of life appears relatively infrequently, and severe RSV infection is rare.[47,53] In Washington, DC, the incidence of RSV infection during the first month of life was noted to be only one third of that during the second month.[8] The protected environment of newborns and their diminished exposure to others may partly explain the lower incidence of illness. Transplacentally derived RSV-specific neutralizing antibody is present in the sera of all term newborns, and may also provide protection from early infection.[8] The level of passive antibody in the term newborn is similar to the maternal level, and gradually declines over the first 6 months of life.

Repeated RSV infections are common in all age groups. Previous infection does not prevent subsequent infections, even in sequential years. In family studies conducted by Glezen et al, RSV infection developed in 69% of children monitored from birth during their first year, and approximately half were reinfected during their second year (Table 1).[5] The rate of reinfection among children who attend day-care is high, as demonstrated by the Chapel Hill studies.[11] These studies showed a 98% initial attack rate among children first exposed to RSV, and reinfection rates in the second and third years of life of 74% and 65%, respectively. After the third infection, disease severity reduced appreciably, suggesting that both age and immune factors are important. It should be noted, however, that because participants in this study were healthy children in day-care centers, the illnesses were relatively mild. Infants with first infections severe enough to require hospitalization rarely appear to have second or repeated infections of equal severity, unless they have an underlying disease that places them at high risk for complications.

Introducing RSV into a family may result in a high attack rate among other family members of all ages.[54] Secondary RSV infection developed in more than 60% of infants and in approximately 40% or more of older children and adults. These infections are usually milder, consisting of tracheobronchitis or an upper respiratory tract infection.[5,55] Children, nevertheless, may experience repeated bouts of RSV lower respiratory tract disease. In preschool children, 20% to more than 50% of the repeated infections involve the lower respiratory tract.[5]

RSV infection in older children is common. In the Tecumseh studies, RSV infection was most frequent in school-aged children.[56] Twenty percent of children 5 to 9 years old were infected during a 1-year period. The rate fell to 10% in family members 15 to 19 years of age, and to 3% to 6% in those 20 to 50 years of age.

RSV causes as much as 4% of community-acquired, lower respiratory tract infections in adults under 60 years of age.[57] Among the elderly, at least 10% of winter hospital admissions are caused by RSV, with a fatality rate of about 10%, similar to that for influenza.[58]

In most adults, RSV infection commonly manifests as an upper respiratory infection (URI). RSV sometimes results in more severe illness, such as bronchitis or an influenza-like condition, especially among parents and hospital staff caring for young infants with RSV infection.[54,59-61] The more severe disease may relate partly to a high-challenge dose from the intimate exposure to infants with primary infection who shed large quantities of virus.[16] Most infections among caregivers, however, are symptomatic, consisting of URI, with or without fever, and tracheobronchitis. In one study, about 70% had an illness more severe and prolonged than the usual 'cold' from other causes.

Little is known about the epidemiology of RSV infection in tropical and developing countries. In most studies, RSV was found to be the cause of acute lower respiratory tract infections in childhood in 27% to 96% of hospitalized viral cases.[9] RSV mostly affects children under 6 months of age in developing countries. Acute lower respiratory tract infections with RSV are slightly more common in boys than in girls. Little information is available about the mortality of children infected with RSV.

Transmission of Infection

RSV usually spreads by close contact with infected people or their infectious secretions, which tend to be profuse, especially in young infants. RSV in nasal secretions of acutely infected infants remains infectious on countertops for more than 6 hours and on cloth and paper tissue for 30 minutes.[62] Furthermore, these nasal secretions remain infectious after transfer from objects or hands to the hands of another person, suggesting that contact with contaminated clothing, furniture, or tissues may be one means of transmission. This mode of spread has been supported by studies demonstrating that infection occurs in volunteers who touch surfaces contaminated by secretions and then touch their eyes or nasal mucosa.[63] In contrast, no infections developed in volunteers exposed to infected infants at a distance of greater than 6 feet, suggesting that small-particle aerosol spread of RSV is not a major transmission mode.

Nosocomial Infection

Nosocomial RSV infection poses a major risk for hospitalized children worldwide, with high infection rates occurring in both infant wards and in neonatal nurseries.[59,64-69] One third or more of nosocomially infected infants have developed pneumonia or bronchiolitis, significantly prolonging their hospital stay.[59] The risk of acquiring nosocomial infection is related to age, underly-

Table 2: Patient Groups at High Risk for Severe RSV Disease

- Premature infants (<35 weeks' gestation)
- Children or adults with chronic lung disease (CLD or bronchopulmonary dysplasia)
- Children with congenital heart disease
- Children or adults with compromised immune function (from chemotherapy, transplant, or congenital or acquired immunodeficiencies)
- Individuals living in institutions
- Elderly people

ing disease, length of hospitalization, and adherence to proper infection-control procedures. Studies in Rochester, NY, show that the proportion of infants hospitalized for other reasons during RSV season who acquire RSV nosocomially varies by year and by infection-control techniques, ranging from 6% to 45%.[59,70]

Nosocomial infection with RSV is also a problem for both adults and children who are immunocompromised.[71,72] During RSV epidemics, infants hospitalized with RSV lower respiratory tract disease pose a hazard to the other young infants admitted with compromising illnesses, and nosocomial infection also occurs on adult wards, threatening immunocompromised patients in that setting.[73-76] Nosocomial infections in immunocompromised children and adults may be particularly serious and difficult to control. Patients hospitalized during the winter months are at great risk of nosocomial RSV infections because RSV is likely to be introduced many times from the community during the season.[77]

Outbreaks on transplant units have been associated with a high mortality rate and prolonged RSV transmission.[78-81]

Table 3: Risk Factors for Acquisition of RSV Infection

- Birth during the months April through September
- Day-care attendance
- Family size
- Crowded living conditions
- Older siblings in school or day-care
- Multiple births
- Lack of breast-feeding

The diagnosis of RSV infection is often not suspected until spread has already occurred. Furthermore, the shedding of RSV from such patients is often abundant and prolonged but may be intermittent. Failing to recognize RSV as a potential nosocomial hazard and failing to employ specific infection-control procedures can result in significant morbidity and mortality.

Hospital staff can readily acquire RSV infection, and may contribute to its spread among patients. Staff may transmit the virus not only by becoming infected and shedding the virus, but also by carrying contaminated secretions on hands, clothing, and objects (such as stethoscopes) to patients.[72,75,82-84] Restricted activity and absenteeism that can affect personnel who have become infected during the RSV season contribute to both the medical and economic costs of RSV infections.

Risk Groups and Risk Factors for Severe RSV Disease

The most severe RSV infections occur among the youngest infants, especially premature infants, and those with bronchopulmonary dysplasia, now called chronic lung disease (CLD). Patients with chronic pulmonary and cardiac diseases, and those with immuno-suppression, are also at high risk for severe RSV infection, with their risk extending well beyond infancy. Institutionalized adults, especially the elderly, are also at risk of complicated disease.

In developed countries, high-risk patients whose RSV infection is likely to progress into severe lower respiratory tract infections are well defined, including adults with chronic underlying disorders and healthy infants younger than 3 months of age. Mortality rates in children in certain risk groups may be as high as 35% to 50%.[51] Certain risk factors have been implicated in more severe disease (Table 2).

Risk factors are not as well defined in developing countries, although crowding, indoor smoke pollution, and malnutrition may play a part in the development of more severe disease. Although the age distribution of RSV in children in developing countries is similar to that seen in developed countries, older children are more seriously affected than those in the developed world, perhaps reflecting these risk factors.[9] A mortality rate of up to 7% has been reported in hospital inpatients in developing countries,[85] much higher than that seen among high-risk patients in developed countries (0.5% to 2.0%). More clinical and epidemiologic studies are required to further define risk factors for severe infection in developing countries.

Patients at Risk for Severe RSV Infection

Premature infants. Prematurity, defined as gestational age less than 36 weeks, with or without correlating CLD, is a risk factor for severe RSV infection, commonly resulting in the need for mechanical ventilation.[86,87] A 1991 study found that 36% of infants with gestational ages of 32 weeks or less required rehospitalization for respiratory illness, compared with 2.5% of term infants.[88] When rehospitalized, preterm infants were compared with preterm infants not requiring rehospitalization; the rehospitalized group had a higher incidence of use of mechanical ventilation and CLD during the neonatal period. The risk of rehospitalization was further increased by discharge from the neonatal intensive care unit (NICU) just before or during the RSV season.

Premature infants with CLD appear to be most at risk for serious illness. Early studies of the risk of rehospitalization for premature infants with CLD estimated that 50% of such children are rehospitalized within 2 years of their initial discharge, primarily because of viral lower respiratory tract infection. In a prospective study of children 2 years or younger with CLD, 59% developed RSV infection, and of these, 69% required hospitalization.[89] Development of RSV disease requiring hospitalization was associated with administration of home oxygen within the previous 3 months. A second study from Denver found that 32% of multiple-birth preterm infants were rehospitalized for RSV, as compared with 18% for singletons.[90] Multiple-birth preterm infants were also at a higher risk for pneumonia than were singletons. Gestational age of less than 30 weeks posed an additional risk factor for developing pneumonia in preterm infants with CLD in this study.

More recent studies have found that premature infants are at less risk of severe RSV disease than previously suggested. Investigators at Kaiser Permanente Northern California found that 3.2% of premature infants in their healthcare system were rehospitalized for RSV.[91] Preterm infants with a lower gestational age (< 32 weeks), a prolonged perinatal oxygen requirement (> 28 days), and NICU discharge within 3 months of the RSV season were most likely to require hospitalization for RSV disease. This study has limitations in that 25% of subjects were lost to follow-up and not all subjects were tested for RSV. In addition, 5% to 10% of infants with duplicate insurance might have been hospitalized elsewhere, and the authors chose to exclude RSV cases presenting in November and April, thus excluding an additional 3% of cases from analysis. A New York study with a 3-year follow-up found that 6.4% of very low birth-weight infants, 2.8% of low birth-weight infants, and 1.7% of normal-weight infants were readmitted with RSV.[92] A third study from Rochester, NY found hospitalization rates of 11.2% for RSV-associated illness for infants born at 32 weeks' gestation or earlier.[93] The incidence of RSV hospitalization increased with decreasing gestational age and was 13.9% for infants born at or before 26 weeks' gestation vs 4.4% for those born at 30 to 32 weeks' gestation.

The duration of risk postdelivery is not well defined. However, a recent small study of 33 premature infants without chronic lung disease suggests that preterm infants remain at risk for severe RSV infection until a postconceptual age of 44 weeks.[94]

Children With Congenital Heart Disease

Infants with congenital heart disease have an increased risk of severe illness from RSV infection. Cyanotic congenital heart disease with left-to-right shunt and pulmonary hypertension has been particularly implicated in severe RSV illness.[95] In a 1980s 5-year prospective study, infants with congenital heart disease hospitalized with RSV during the first year of life required intensive care 4 times more often than normal infants. The mortality rate for infants with congenital heart disease was 37%, compared with 1.5% for infants without underlying disease.[95] More recent studies find that RSV mortality rates in pediatric patients with congenital heart disease are 2.5% to 3.5%.[96,97] RSV infection in congenital heart disease patients with pulmonary hypertension has been associated with increased morbidity (increased hospital days and greater intensive care and mechanical ventilation durations) but not increased mortality rates. The markedly decreased mortality risk from RSV infection in patients with congenital heart disease is likely caused by improvements in intensive care management and advances in surgical cardiac correction.

RSV is not only a problem for children with underlying cardiac disease, it is also a risk factor for those undergoing cardiac surgery during RSV season. Cardiac surgery performed during the symptomatic period of RSV infection is associated with a higher rate of postoperative complications, especially postoperative pulmonary hypertension. These complications appear more frequently and more severely in patients who had surgery during the course of their RSV infection compared with those who had surgery after the infection resolved.[98]

Young Children With Chronic Pulmonary Conditions

Children with significant pulmonary compromise are at risk of more severe RSV infection than other children. The PICNIC group compared outcomes of RSV infection in children with CLD to those with other pulmonary disorders, such as cystic fibrosis, recurrent aspiration pneumonitis, pulmonary malformation, neurogenic disorders interfering with pulmonary toilet, and tracheoesophageal fistula, hospitalized at Canadian pediatric hospitals from 1993 through 1995. Regardless of the underlying condition, the duration of hospitalization, ICU admission, duration of ICU stay, mechanical ventilation, and duration of mechanical ventilation, the outcomes were similar.[99] The use of home oxygen was associated with a greater risk of ICU admission regardless of underlying diagnosis.[99]

RSV infections may be prolonged in infants with cystic fibrosis when compared to otherwise healthy infants. RSV episodes may also contribute to the chronic lung damage and accelerate the pulmonary deterioration of patients with cystic fibrosis.[100]

Older Children and Adults With Chronic Pulmonary Conditions

RSV has been increasingly recognized as causing serious respiratory illness in adults with underlying cardiopulmonary disease.[101] Several studies have been undertaken to estimate the clinical impact of RSV infection in patients with chronic underlying conditions. Glezen et al, in a survey of viral etiology of patients hospitalized with acute respiratory tract conditions between July 1991 and June 1995, found that 93% of patients older than 5 years had a chronic underlying condition, with chronic pulmonary conditions most common.[102] In addition, patients with chronic pulmonary disease from low-income populations were hospitalized at a rate almost 8 times that of patients from middle-income groups. Influenza, parainfluenza, and RSV infections accounted for 75% of all virus infections. Walsh found the clinical illnesses associated with RSV in persons with chronic obstructive pulmonary disease (COPD) and congestive heart failure residing in the community were similar to those with influenza A virus.[103] Thirty-seven percent of RSV-infected subjects were hospitalized.

Immunocompromised Children and Adults

RSV frequently causes respiratory illness and is associated with high rates of morbidity and mortality among immunocompromised patients.[104] Infants and children with congenital, acquired, or chemotherapeutically induced states of immunodeficiency with major impairment of T-cell function are at high risk for development of severe and prolonged bronchopulmonary disease, and in some instances, for the development of giant cell pneumonia and extramucosal spread of the virus. Although fatalities have been reported in immunocompromised RSV-infected infants and children, the extent of morbidity or mortality directly related to RSV in such patients is unknown.[105,106]

For infants and children undergoing chemotherapy for underlying malignancies, RSV infection poses a serious problem, with significantly increased and prolonged virus shedding and possible development of severe lower respiratory tract disease.[107] Severe disease with increased morbidity has also been observed during and after immunosuppressive therapy in older patients ranging in age from 3 to 40 years.[78,96,108]

Available data on RSV infection in congenital forms of severe immunodeficiency diseases are limited to only a few studies, primarily of patients with severe combined immunodeficiency syndrome.[109-113] Most patients studied have had pronounced pulmonary disease or giant cell pneumonia, with prolonged virus shedding (more than 100 days in some cases). Although cases of severe or fatal RSV infection have been observed in patients with AIDS, most HIV-infected children have illnesses that are similar to non-HIV-infected children, with the exception of more prolonged shedding of RSV.[114-116]

Patients receiving corticosteroids alone do not appear to be at the same level of increased risk for severe disease as other immunocompromised patient groups. Steroid treatment, however, seems to increase the quantity of viral shedding.[106]

RSV infections cause significant morbidity and mortality in both adult and pediatric bone marrow and solid organ transplant recipients.[78,113,117-119] Adult bone marrow recipients may have severe and even fatal disease, especially when infection occurs before marrow engraftment.[74,78,79] RSV infection occurring soon after solid organ transplantation may also be severe.[120] In contrast to other solid organ transplant recipients, RSV is rarely isolated from adult recipients after liver transplantation and the illness is somewhat modified.[121] Several abstracts suggest that liver transplant patients have severe and even fatal disease if they contract RSV in the month immediately after transplant surgery when the patient is still on immunosuppresive therapy.

Elderly Patients and Institutionalized Adults

RSV is increasingly recognized as a cause of serious disease in older adults. RSV causes disease that may clini-

Table 4: Host-related Factors Increasing Severity of RSV Infection

- Age <6 months
- Premature birth
- Multiple gestation
- Male gender
- Low socioeconomic status
- Crowded living conditions
- Indoor smoke pollution
- Malnutrition
- Family history of atopy or asthma
- Lower cord serum antibody titers

cally be indistinguishable from influenza, and also causes excessive morbidity and mortality in older persons residing in nursing homes and in the community.[122,123] In the United States, 687,000 hospitalizations and 74,000 deaths caused by pneumonia occur annually among the elderly; 2% to 9% of these are caused by RSV.[124] RSV infection may result in death as often as influenza.[125] From 1988 to 1999, Drinka studied nursing home residents and found that mortality following isolation of RSV was 4%, comparable to that following influenza A.[126] Results of studies by Falsey et al suggest that older adults with low titers of serum-neutralizing antibody may be at greater risk of developing symptomatic RSV infection than those who have high antibody titers.[127]

Severe RSV-related illness also occurs in institutionalized young adults.[128] Although most RSV infections involved the upper respiratory tract only, severe RSV infection was seen in 17% of the young adult residents in an institution for the developmentally disabled in 1 study, and 1 patient died of severe bronchopneumonia.

Risk Factors for Acquisition of RSV

Risk factors for acquiring RSV bronchiolitis in infants and young children identified in epidemiologic studies in the United States include: birth between April and the end of September, day-care attendance, lack of breast-feeding, residence in crowded homes, multiple births, and more siblings[53,129] (Table 3). Many of the factors that increase the risk of RSV, such as family size, siblings in school, or day-care, increase the likelihood of being infected at a young age, thereby increasing the risk of lower respiratory tract disease in association with infection.

Day-care Attendance

RSV infection rates among children who attend day-care is high, as demonstrated by the Chapel Hill studies.[11] These studies showed a 98% initial attack rate among children first exposed to RSV in the day-care setting. A study by Anderson also found that day-care was an important risk factor for acquiring lower respiratory tract illness in children less than 2 years of age.[130]

Family Size

RSV spreads effectively through exposed families, and the virus is most commonly introduced through a school-age child.[54,56,131,132] Disease in an infant is likely to follow an older sibling's mild 'cold.'[59] A prospective study of families that included an infant and 1 or more older siblings showed that 44% of the families became infected with RSV during a 3-month epidemic. In most of these families, older siblings (2 to 16 years of age) introduced the virus into the family, and the infants became infected secondarily. Furthermore, intrafamilial spread of the virus, according to the Tecumseh study, was related to the number of family members.[56] Families with 6 members had approximately 3 times the rate of infection than that observed in families of 3. In studies of premature infants, family size of 4 or more people was an important factor predictive of acquiring an RSV infection.[89,90] Twins and triplets are also at greater risk for RSV infection and more severe RSV disease.[90]

Breast-feeding

Studies on the effect of breast-feeding on RSV infection have been inconclusive. Some suggest that breast-feeding is protective,[133,134] while others found no benefit in preventing respiratory viral infections.[130,135,136]

Risk Factors for Increased Severity of Infection in Healthy Infants and Children

Risk factors identified with increased severity of RSV infection in healthy infants and children include male gender, low socioeconomic status, crowded living conditions, indoor smoke pollution, malnutrition, a family history of asthma or atopy, and lower cord serum RSV antibody titers (Table 4).

Gender

According to most studies of children hospitalized with RSV disease, males predominate in a ratio of about 2 to 1.[8,137] However, in children with milder RSV illness, boys and girls are equally affected, suggesting that gender influences the expression rather than the rate of illness, with boys developing more severe disease.[16,55]

Socioeconomic Status

Infants from more affluent socioeconomic environments tend to be older when they first acquire lower respiratory tract disease from RSV, and less frequently have severe disease.[138] In a private practice in Chapel Hill, only 13% of the bronchiolitis patients were younger than 6 months of age, compared with 40% in the day-care center, and 56% of hospitalized cases.[55] The risk of hospitalization with RSV disease for infants from middle-income families in Chapel Hill was less than 1 per 1,000, compared with a 5- to 10-fold greater risk for infants of low-income families in Houston and Washington, DC.[5,10,16,40,47] Similarly, rates of hospitalization for RSV disease have been lower in children from middle-income families in Seattle and from a less-urban area in Michigan.[19,56] Crowding and unemployment also seem to increase the incidence of hospital admission in England.[44,45] In the city of Tyneside, 1 of every 50 infants required hospital admission for RSV infection during the first year of life.

Air Pollution and Smoking

Passive exposure to environmental air contamination increases the risk of severe RSV infection. Epidemiologic studies link increased pulmonary morbidity with RSV infection to episodes of high-particulate air pollution.[139] Several studies also suggest that exposure to cigarette smoke is a risk factor for RSV lower respiratory tract infection in infants.[6,89,136,140,141]

Malnutrition

Viral respiratory infection in protein-calorie deprived mice has been associated with defects in cell-mediated immunity and with more severe disease in the malnourished animals.[142,143] Malnutrition and vitamin A deficiency are risk factors for severe RSV infection requiring hospitalization in some developing countries.[139,144]

Family History of Asthma or Atopy

Family history of asthma or atopy can possibly increase the risk for RSV-related lower respiratory tract illness. Some studies demonstrate significantly higher rates of severe RSV infection in children with atopy compared with control children,[145,146] while other studies show no significant association.[129,136,147] Diminished lung function may be a predisposing factor for lower respiratory tract infection associated with wheezing.[148]

Low Anti-RSV Antibody Titers

Holberg et al demonstrated that infants with lower cord serum RSV antibody, who also received minimal breast-feeding, were found to be especially at risk for RSV lower respiratory tract infections during the first 5 months of life.[53] This phenomenon was also observed in Alaskan Native infants where RSV microneutralizing antibody titers <1,200 were associated with severe disease.[149] Low or absent RSV antibody titers also appear to play an important role in the development of severe RSV disease observed in preterm infants.[86,89]

Summary

RSV is a major cause of viral lower respiratory tract infections among infants and young children in both developing and developed countries, an important cause of disease in adults, and is responsible for significant morbidity and mortality in the elderly. It can also be devastating in immunosuppressed populations. RSV infects most children by the time they are 2 years old and reinfects throughout life. RSV is best recognized for causing bronchiolitis in infants.

The most severe infections with RSV occur in the youngest infants, especially premature infants and those with chronic lung disease. Patients with chronic pulmonary and cardiac diseases and those with immunosuppression also are at high risk for severe RSV infection, and their risk may last well beyond infancy. Institutionalized adults, especially the elderly, are also at risk of complicated disease. Understanding the natural history of RSV infection, the burden of disease attributable to RSV, and the risk factors for severe RSV infection is vital for the development of strategies for treatment and prevention of RSV.

References

1. Garenne M, Ronsmans C, Campbell H: The magnitude of mortality from acute respiratory infections in children under 5 years in developing countries. *World Health Stat Q* 1992;45:180-191.

2.   Institute of Medicine: The prospects for immunizing against respiratory syncytial virus. New vaccine development, establishing priorities. In: *Diseases of Importance in the United States.* Washington, DC, National Academy Press, 1985, pp 397-409.

3.   Berman S: Epidemiology of acute respiratory infections in children of developing countries. *Rev Infect Dis* 1991;13(suppl 6):S454-S462.

4.   Glezen P, Denny FW: Epidemiology of acute lower respiratory disease in children. *N Engl J Med* 1973;288:498-505.

5.   Glezen WP, Taber LH, Frank AL, et al: Risk of primary infection and reinfection with respiratory syncytial virus. *Am J Dis Child* 1986;140:543-546.

6.   Hayes EB, Hurwitz ES, Schonberger LB, et al: Respiratory syncytial virus outbreak on American Samoa. Evaluation of risk factors. *Am J Dis Child* 1989;143:316-321.

7.   Morrell RE, Marks MI, Champlin R, et al: An outbreak of severe pneumonia due to respiratory syncytial virus in isolated Arctic populations. *Am J Epidemiol* 1975;101:231-237.

8.   Parrott RH, Kim HW, Arrobio JO, et al: Epidemiology of respiratory syncytial virus infection in Washington, D.C. II. Infection and disease with respect to age, immunologic status, race and sex. *Am J Epidemiol* 1973;98:289-300.

9.   Weber MW, Mulholland EK, Greenwood BM: Respiratory syncytial virus infection in tropical and developing countries. *Trop Med Int Health* 1998;3:268-280.

10.   Kim HW, Arrobio JO, Brandt CD, et al: Epidemiology of respiratory syncytial virus infection in Washington, D.C. I. Importance of the virus in different respiratory tract disease syndromes and temporal distribution of infection. *Am J Epidemiol* 1973;98:216-225.

11.   Henderson FW, Collier AM, Clyde WA Jr, et al: Respiratory-syncytial-virus infections, reinfections and immunity. A prospective, longitudinal study in young children. *N Engl J Med* 1979;300:530-534.

12.   Update: respiratory syncytial virus activity—United States, 1998-1999 season. *MMWR Morb Mortal Wkly Rep* 1999;48:1104-1106, 1115.

13. Halstead DC, Jenkins SG: Continuous non-seasonal epidemic of respiratory syncytial virus infection in the southeast United States. *South Med J* 1998;91:433-436.

14. Update: respiratory syncytial virus activity—United States, 1997-98 season. *MMWR Morb Mortal Wkly Rep* 1997;46:1163-1165.

15. Chew FT, Doraisingham S, Ling AE, et al: Seasonal trends of viral respiratory tract infections in the tropics. *Epidemiol Infect* 1998;121:121-128.

16. Glezen WP: Pathogenesis of bronchiolitis—epidemiologic considerations. *Pediatr Res* 1977;11:239-243.

17. Mufson MA, Levine HD, Wasil RE, et al: Epidemiology of respiratory syncytial virus infection among infants and children in Chicago. *Am J Epidemiol* 1973;98:88-95.

18. Hall C, McBride J: Bronchiolitis. In: Mandell, ed. *Principles and Practice of Infectious Diseases*. New York, NY, Churchill Livingstone Inc, 1999.

19. Foy HM, Cooney MK, Maletzky AJ, et al: Incidence and etiology of pneumonia, croup and bronchiolitis in preschool children belonging to a prepaid medical care group over a four-year period. *Am J Epidemiol* 1973;97:80-92.

20. Hall CB, Walsh EE, Schnabel KC, et al: Occurrence of groups A and B of respiratory syncytial virus over 15 years: associated epidemiologic and clinical characteristics in hospitalized and ambulatory children. *J Infect Dis* 1990;162:1283-1290.

21. Sullender WM: Respiratory syncytial virus genetic and antigenic diversity. *Clin Microbiol Rev* 2000;13:1-15.

22. Akerlind B, Norrby E: Occurrence of respiratory syncytial virus subtypes A and B strains in Sweden. *J Med Virol* 1986;19:241-247.

23. Anderson LJ, Hendry RM, Pierik LT, et al: Multicenter study of strains of respiratory syncytial virus. *J Infect Dis* 1991;163:687-692.

24. Hendry RM, Talis AL, Godfrey E, et al: Concurrent circulation of antigenically distinct strains of respiratory syncytial virus during community outbreaks. *J Infect Dis* 1986;153:291-297.

25. Hendry RM, Pierik LT, McIntosh K: Prevalence of respiratory syncytial virus subgroups over six consecutive outbreaks: 1981-1987. *J Infect Dis* 1989;160:185-190.

26. Mufson MA, Belshe RB, Orvell C, et al: Respiratory syncytial virus epidemics: variable dominance of subgroups A and B strains among children, 1981-1986. *J Infect Dis* 1988;157:143-148.

27. Mufson MA, Akerlind-Stopner B, Orvell C, et al: A single-season epidemic with respiratory syncytial virus subgroup B2 during 10 epidemic years, 1978 to 1988. *J Clin Microbiol* 1991;29:162-165.

28. Storch GA, Anderson LJ, Park CS, et al: Antigenic and genomic diversity within group A respiratory syncytial virus. *J Infect Dis* 1991;163:858-861.

29. Tsutsumi H, Onuma M, Suga K, et al: Occurrence of respiratory syncytial virus subgroup A and B strains in Japan, 1980 to 1987. *J Clin Microbiol* 1988;26:1171-1174.

30. Peret TC, Hall CB, Schnabel KC, et al: Circulation patterns of genetically distinct group A and B strains of human respiratory syncytial virus in a community. *J Gen Virol* 1998;79:2221-2229.

31. Taylor CE, Morrow S, Scott M, et al: Comparative virulence of respiratory syncytial virus subgroups A and B. *Lancet* 1989;1:777-778.

32. Freymuth F, Petitjean J, Pothier P, et al: Prevalence of respiratory syncytial virus subgroups A and B in France from 1982 to 1990. *J Clin Microbiol* 1991;29:653-655.

33. Anderson LJ, Heilman CA: Protective and disease-enhancing immune responses to respiratory syncytial virus. *J Infect Dis* 1995;171:1-7.

34. Mufson MA, Belshe RB, Orvell C, et al: Subgroup characteristics of respiratory syncytial virus strains recovered from children with two consecutive infections. *J Clin Microbiol* 1987;25:1535-1539.

35. Waris M: Pattern of respiratory syncytial virus epidemics in Finland: two-year cycles with alternating prevalence of groups A and B. *J Infect Dis* 1991;163:464-469.

36. McConnochie KM, Hall CB, Walsh EE, et al: Variation in severity of respiratory syncytial virus infections with subtype. *J Pediatr* 1990;117:52-62.

37. Walsh EE, McConnochie KM, Long CE, et al: Severity of respiratory syncytial virus infection is related to virus strain. *J Infect Dis* 1997;175:814-820.

38. Parrott RH, Kim HW, Brandt CD, et al: Respiratory syncytial virus in infants and children. *Prev Med* 1974;3:473-480.

39. Heilman C: From the National Institute of Allergy and Infectious Diseases and the World Health Organization. Respiratory syncytial and parainfluenza viruses. *J Infect Dis* 1990;161:402-406.

40. Henderson FW, Clyde WA Jr, Collier AM, et al: The etiologic and epidemiologic spectrum of bronchiolitis in pediatric practice. *J Pediatr* 1979;95:183-190.

41. Murphy TF, Henderson FW, Clyde WA Jr, et al: Pneumonia: an eleven-year study in a pediatric practice. *Am J Epidemiol* 1981;113:12-21.

42. Loda FA, Clyde WA Jr, Glezen WP, et al: Studies on the role of viruses, bacteria, and *M pneumoniae* as causes of lower respiratory tract infections in children. *J Pediatr* 1968;72:161-176.

43. Foy HM, Cooney MK, McMahan R, et al: Viral and mycoplasmal pneumonia in a prepaid medical care group during an eight-year period. *Am J Epidemiol* 1973;97:93-102.

44. Sims DG, Downham MA, McQuillin J, et al: Respiratory syncytial virus infection in north-east England. *Br Med J* 1976;2:1095-1098.

45. Respiratory syncytial virus infection: admissions to hospital in industrial, urban, and rural areas. Report to the Medical Research Council Subcommittee on Respiratory Syncytial Virus Vaccines. *Br Med J* 1978;2:796-798.

46. Denny FW, Clyde WA Jr: Acute lower respiratory tract infections in nonhospitalized children. *J Pediatr* 1986;108:635-646.

47. Glezen WP, Paredes A, Allison JE, et al: Risk of respiratory syncytial virus infection for infants from low-income families in relationship to age, sex, ethnic group, and maternal antibody level. *J Pediatr* 1981;98:708-715.

48. McConnochie KM, Roghmann KJ: Parental smoking, presence of older siblings, and family history of asthma increase risk of bronchiolitis. *Am J Dis Child* 1986;140:806-812.

49. Wright AL, Taussig LM, Ray CG, et al: The Tucson Children's Respiratory Study. II. Lower respiratory tract illness in the first year of life. *Am J Epidemiol* 1989;129:1232-1246.

50. Shay DK, Holman RC, Newman RD, et al: Bronchiolitis-associated hospitalizations among US children, 1980-1996. *JAMA* 1999;282:1440-1446.

51. McIntosh K: Respiratory syncytial virus infections in infants and children: diagnosis and treatment. *Pediatr Rev* 1987;9:191-196.

52. Hall CB: Respiratory syncytial virus. In: Feigin RD, Cherry JD, eds. *Textbook of Pediatric Infectious Diseases*, 4th ed. Philadelphia, WB Saunders Co, 1998, pp 2084-2111.

53. Holberg CJ, Wright AL, Martinez FD, et al: Risk factors for respiratory syncytial virus-associated lower respiratory illnesses in the first year of life. *Am J Epidemiol* 1991;133:1135-1151.

54. Hall CB, Geiman JM, Biggar R, et al: Respiratory syncytial virus infections within families. *N Engl J Med* 1976;294:414-419.

55. Denny FW, Collier AM, Henderson FW, et al: The epidemiology of bronchiolitis. *Pediatr Res* 1977;11:234-236.

56. Monto AS, Lim SK: The Tecumseh study of respiratory illness. III. Incidence and periodicity of respiratory syncytial virus and *Mycoplasma pneumoniae* infections. *Am J Epidemiol* 1971;94:290-301.

57. Dowell SF, Anderson LJ, Gary HE Jr, et al: Respiratory syncytial virus is an important cause of community-acquired lower respiratory infection among hospitalized adults. *J Infect Dis* 1996;174:456-462.

58. Falsey AR, Cunningham CK, Barker WH, et al: Respiratory syncytial virus and influenza A infections in the hospitalized elderly. *J Infect Dis* 1995;172:389-394.

59. Hall CB, Douglas RG Jr, Geiman JM, et al: Nosocomial respiratory syncytial virus infections. *N Engl J Med* 1975;293:1343-1346.

60. Hall WJ, Hall CB, Speers DM: Respiratory syncytial virus infection in adults: clinical, virologic, and serial pulmonary function studies. *Ann Intern Med* 1978;88:203-205.

61. Hall CB, Walsh EE, Long CE, et al: Immunity to and frequency of reinfection with respiratory syncytial virus. *J Infect Dis* 1991;163:693-698.

62. Hall CB, Douglas RG Jr, Geiman JM: Possible transmission by fomites of respiratory syncytial virus. *J Infect Dis* 1980;141:98-102.

63. Hall CB, Douglas RG Jr: Modes of transmission of respiratory syncytial virus. *J Pediatr* 1981;99:100-103.

64. Ditchburn RK, McQuillin J, Gardner PS, et al: Respiratory syncytial virus in hospital cross-infection. *Br Med J* 1971;3:671-673.

65. Donowitz LG: Hospital-acquired infections in children. *N Engl J Med* 1990;323:1836-1837.

66. Gardner PS, Court SD, Brocklebank JT, et al: Virus cross-infection in paediatric wards. *Br Med J* 1973;2:571-575.

67. Hall CB: The shedding and spreading of respiratory syncytial virus. *Pediatr Res* 1977;11:236-239.

68. Meissner HC, Murray SA, Kiernan MA, et al: A simultaneous outbreak of respiratory syncytial virus and parainfluenza virus type 3 in a newborn nursery. *J Pediatr* 1984;104:680-684.

69. Sims DG, Downham MA, Webb JK, et al: Hospital cross-infection on children's wards with respiratory syncytial virus and the role of adult carriage. *Acta Paediatr Scand* 1975;64:541-645.

70. Hall CB, Powell KR, Schnabel KC, et al: Risk of secondary bacterial infection in infants hospitalized with respiratory syncytial viral infection. *J Pediatr* 1988;113:266-271.

71. Landry ML: Multiple viral infections in the immunocompromised host: recognition and interpretation. *Clin Diagn Virol* 1994;2:313-321.

72. Nosocomial infection with respiratory syncytial virus. *Lancet* 1992;340:1071-1073.

73. Guidry GG, Black-Payne CA, Payne DK, et al: Respiratory syncytial virus infection among intubated adults in a university medical intensive care unit. *Chest* 1991;100:1377-1384.

74. Hertz MI, Englund JA, Snover D, et al: Respiratory syncytial virus-induced acute lung injury in adult patients with bone marrow transplants: a clinical approach and review of the literature. *Medicine* 1989;68:269-281.

75. Whimbey E, Bodey GP: Viral pneumonia in the immunocompromised adult with neoplastic disease: the role of common community respiratory viruses. *Semin Respir Infect* 1992;7:122-131.

76. Takimoto CH, Cram DL, Root RK: Respiratory syncytial virus infections on an adult medical ward. *Arch Intern Med* 1991;151:706-708.

77. Mazzulli T, Peret T, McGeer A, et al: Molecular characterization of a nosocomial outbreak of human respiratory syncytial virus on an adult leukemia/lymphoma ward. *J Infect Dis* 1999;180:1686-1689.

78. Englund JA, Sullivan CJ, Jordan MC, et al: Respiratory syncytial virus infection in immunocompromised adults. *Ann Intern Med* 1988;109:203-208.

79. Harrington RD, Hooton TM, Hackman RC, et al: An outbreak of respiratory syncytial virus in a bone marrow transplant center. *J Infect Dis* 1992;165:987-993.

80. Jones BL, Clark S, Curran ET, et al: Control of an outbreak of respiratory syncytial virus infection in immunocompromised adults. *J Hosp Infect* 2000;44:53-57.

81. Tolkoff-Rubin NE, Rubin H: New strategies for the control of viral infection in organ transplantation. *Clin Transplant* 1995;9:255-259.

82. Goldmann DA: Transmission of infectious diseases in children. *Pediatr Rev* 1992;13:283-293.

83. Hall CB: The nosocomial spread of respiratory syncytial viral infections. *Annu Rev Med* 1983;34:311-319.

84. Agah R, Cherry JD, Garakian AJ, et al: Respiratory syncytial virus (RSV) infection rate in personnel caring for children with RSV infections. Routine isolation procedure vs routine procedure supplemented by use of masks and goggles. *Am J Dis Child* 1987;141:695-697.

85. Cherian T, Simoes EA, Steinhoff MC, et al: Bronchiolitis in tropical south India. *Am J Dis Child* 1990;144:1026-1030.

86. Meert K, Heidemann S, Abella B, et al: Does prematurity alter the course of respiratory syncytial virus infection? *Crit Care Med* 1990;18:1357-1359.

87. Wang EE, Law BJ, Stephens D: Pediatric Investigators Collaborative Network on Infections in Canada (PICNIC) prospective study of risk factors and outcomes in patients hospitalized with respiratory syncytial viral lower respiratory tract infection. *J Pediatr* 1995;126:212-219.

88. Cunningham CK, McMillan JA, Gross SJ: Rehospitalization for respiratory illness in infants of less than 32 weeks' gestation. *Pediatrics* 1991;88:527-532.

89. Groothuis JR, Gutierrez KM, Lauer BA: Respiratory syncytial virus infection in children with bronchopulmonary dysplasia. *Pediatrics* 1988;82:199-203.

90. Simoes EA, King SJ, Lehr MV, et al: Preterm twins and triplets. A high-risk group for severe respiratory syncytial virus infection. *Am J Dis Child* 1993;147:303-306.

91. Joffe S, Escobar GJ, Black SB, et al: Rehospitalization for respiratory syncytial virus among premature infants. *Pediatrics* 1999;104:894-899.

92. Nachman SA, Navaie-Waliser M, Qureshi MZ: Rehospitalization with respiratory syncytial virus after neonatal intensive care unit discharge: A 3-year follow-up. *Pediatrics* 1997;100:E8.

93. Stevens TP, Sinkin RA, Hall CB, et al: Respiratory syncytial virus and premature infants born at 32 weeks' gestation or earlier: hospitalization and economic implications of prophylaxis. *Arch Pediatr Adolesc Med* 2000;154:55-61.

94. Bont L, van Vught AJ, Kimpen JL: Prophylaxis against respiratory syncytial virus in premature infants. *Lancet* 1999;354:1003-1004.

95. MacDonald N, Hall C, Suffin S, et al: Respiratory syncytial viral infection in infants with congenital heart disease. *N Engl J Med* 1982;307:397-400.

96. Navas L, Wang E, de Carvalho V, et al: Improved outcome of respiratory syncytial virus infection in a high-risk hospitalized population of Canadian children. Pediatric Investigators Collaborative Network on Infections in Canada. *J Pediatr* 1992;121:348-354.

97. Moler FW, Khan AS, Meliones JN, et al: Respiratory syncytial virus morbidity and mortality estimates in congenital heart disease patients: a recent experience. *Crit Care Med* 1992;20:1406-1413.

98. Khongphatthanayothin A, Wong PC, Samara Y, et al: Impact of respiratory syncytial virus infection on surgery for congenital heart disease: postoperative course and outcome. *Crit Care Med* 1999;27:1974-1981.

99. Arnold SR, Wang EE, Law BJ, et al: Variable morbidity of respiratory syncytial virus infection in patients with underlying lung disease: a review of the PICNIC RSV database. Pediatric Investigators Collaborative Network on Infections in Canada. *Pediatr Infect Dis J* 1999;18:866-869.

100. Abman SH, Ogle JW, Butler-Simon N, et al: Role of respiratory syncytial virus in early hospitalizations for respiratory distress of young infants with cystic fibrosis. *J Pediatr* 1988;113:826-830.

101. Yang E, Rubin BK: 'Childhood' viruses as a cause of pneumonia in adults. *Semin Respir Infect* 1995;10:232-243.

102. Glezen WP, Greenberg SB, Atmar RL, et al: Impact of respiratory virus infections on persons with chronic underlying conditions. *JAMA* 2000;283:499-505.

103. Walsh EE, Falsey AR, Hennessey PA: Respiratory syncytial and other virus infections in persons with chronic cardiopulmonary disease. *Am J Respir Crit Care Med* 1999;160:791-795.

104. Rabella N, Rodriguez P, Labeaga R, et al: Conventional respiratory viruses recovered from immunocompromised patients: clinical considerations. *Clin Infect Dis* 1999;28:1043-1048.

105. Fishaut M, Tubergen D, McIntosh K: Cellular response to respiratory viruses with particular reference to children with disorders of cell-mediated immunity. *J Pediatr* 1980;96:179-186.

106. Hall CB, Powell KR, MacDonald NE, et al: Respiratory syncytial viral infection in children with compromised immune function. *N Engl J Med* 1986;315:77-81.

107. Craft AW, Reid MM, Gardner PS, et al: Virus infections in children with acute lymphoblastic leukaemia. *Arch Dis Child* 1979;54:755-759.

108. Englund JA, Anderson LJ, Rhame FS: Nosocomial transmission of respiratory syncytial virus in immunocompromised adults. *J Clin Microbiol* 1991;29:115-119.

109. Delage G, Brochu P, Robillard L, et al: Giant cell pneumonia due to respiratory syncytial virus. Occurrence in severe combined immunodeficiency syndrome. *Arch Pathol Lab Med* 1984;108:623-625.

110. McIntosh K, Kurachek SC, Cairns LM, et al: Treatment of respiratory viral infection in an immunodeficient infant with ribavirin aerosol. *Am J Dis Child* 1984;138:305-308.

111. Milner ME, de la Monte SM, Hutchins GM: Fatal respiratory syncytial virus infection in severe combined immunodeficiency syndrome. *Am J Dis Child* 1985;139:1111-1114.

112. Schneider S, Borzy MS: Fatal respiratory syncytial virus pneumonia as the presenting feature of severe combined immunodeficiency disease. *Clin Pediatr (Phila)* 1996;35:147-149.

113. Taylor CE, Osman HK, Turner AJ, et al: Parainfluenza virus and respiratory syncytial virus infection in infants undergoing bone

marrow transplantation for severe combined immunodeficiency. *Commun Dis Public Health* 1998;1:202-203.

114. Wallace JM: Pulmonary infection in human immunodeficiency disease: viral pulmonary infections. *Semin Respir Infect* 1989;4:147-154.

115. King JC Jr, Burke AR, Clemens JD, et al: Respiratory syncytial virus illnesses in human immunodeficiency virus- and noninfected children. *Pediatr Infect Dis J* 1993;12:733-739.

116. Chandwani S, Borkowsky W, Krasinski K, et al: Respiratory syncytial virus infection in human immunodeficiency virus-infected children. *J Pediatr* 1990;117:251-254.

117. Anderson DJ, Jordan MC: Viral pneumonia in recipients of solid organ transplants. *Semin Respir Infect* 1990;5:38-49.

118. Palmer S Jr, Henshaw NG, Howell DN, et al: Community respiratory viral infection in adult lung transplant recipients. *Chest* 1998;113:944-950.

119. Garcia R, Raad I, Abi-Said D, et al: Nosocomial respiratory syncytial virus infections: prevention and control in bone marrow transplant patients. *Infect Control Hosp Epidemiol* 1997;18:412-416.

120. Pohl C, Green M, Wald ER, et al: Respiratory syncytial virus infections in pediatric liver transplant recipients. *J Infect Dis* 1992;165:166-169.

121. Singhal S, Muir D, Ratcliffe D, et al: Respiratory viruses in adult liver transplant recipients. *Transplantation* 1999;68:981-984.

122. Falsey AR: Respiratory syncytial virus infection in older persons. *Vaccine* 1998;16:1775-1778.

123. Nicholson K, Kent J, Hammersley V, et al: Acute viral infections of upper respiratory tract in elderly people living in the community: comparative, prospective, population-based study of disease burden. *BMJ* 1997;315:1060-1064.

124. Han L, Alexander JP, Anderson LJ: Respiratory syncytial virus pneumonia among the elderly: an assessment of disease burden. *J Infect Dis* 1999;179:25-30.

125. Crowcroft NS, Cutts F, Zambon MC: Respiratory syncytial virus: an underestimated cause of respiratory infection, with prospects for a vaccine. *Commun Dis Public Health* 1999;2:234-241.

126. Drinka P, Gravenstein S, Langer E, et al: Mortality following isolation of various respiratory viruses in nursing home residents. *Infect Control Hosp Epidemiol* 1999;20:812-815.

127. Falsey AR, Walsh EE: Relationship of serum antibody to risk of respiratory syncytial virus infection in elderly adults. *J Infect Dis* 1998;177:463-466.

128. Finger R, Anderson LJ, Dicker RC, et al: Epidemic infections caused by respiratory syncytial virus in institutionalized young adults. *J Infect Dis* 1987;155:1335-1339.

129. Carlsen KH, Larsen S, Bjerve O, et al: Acute bronchiolitis: predisposing factors and characterization of infants at risk. *Pediatr Pulmonol* 1987;3:153-160.

130. Anderson LJ, Parker RA, Strikas RA, et al: Day-care center attendance and hospitalization for lower respiratory tract illness. *Pediatrics* 1988;82:300-308.

131. Berglund B: Respiratory syncytial virus infections in families. A study of family members of children hospitalized for acute respiratory disease. *Acta Paediatr Scand* 1967;56:395-404.

132. Monto AS, Cavallaro JJ: The Tecumseh study of respiratory illness. II. Patterns of occurrence of infection with respiratory pathogens, 1965-1969. *Am J Epidemiol* 1971;94:280-289.

133. Downham MA, Scott R, Sims DG, et al: Breast-feeding protects against respiratory syncytial virus infections. *Br Med J* 1976;2:274-276.

134. Pullan CR, Toms GL, Martin AJ, et al: Breast-feeding and respiratory syncytial virus infection. *Br Med J* 1980;281:1034-1036.

135. Videla C, Carballal G, Misirlian A, et al: Acute lower respiratory infections due to respiratory syncytial virus and adenovirus among hospitalized children from Argentina. *Clin Diagn Virol* 1998;10:17-23.

136. Hall CB, Hall WJ, Gala CL, et al: Long-term prospective study in children after respiratory syncytial virus infection. *J Pediatr* 1984;105:358-364.

137. Hall CB, Douglas RG Jr: Clinically useful method for the isolation of respiratory syncytial virus. *J Infect Dis* 1975;131:1-5.

138. McConnochie KM, Hall CB, Barker WH: Lower respiratory tract illness in the first two years of life: epidemiologic patterns and costs in a suburban pediatric practice. *Am J Public Health* 1988;78:34-39.

139. Vardas E, Blaauw D, McAnerney J: The epidemiology of respiratory syncytial virus (RSV) infections in South African children. *S Afr Med J* 1999;89:1079-1084.

140. Harlap S, Davies AM: Infant admissions to hospital and maternal smoking. *Lancet* 1974;1:529-532.

141. Sims DG, Downham MA, Gardner PS, et al: Study of 8-year-old children with a history of respiratory syncytial virus bronchiolitis in infancy. *Br Med J* 1978;1:11-14.

142. Pena-Cruz V, Reiss CS, McIntosh K: Sendai virus infection of mice with protein malnutrition. *J Virol* 1989;63:3541-3544.

143. Pena-Cruz V, Reiss C, McIntosh K: Effect of respiratory syncytial virus infection on mice with protein malnutrition. *J Med Virol* 1991;33:219-223.

144. Dowell SF, Papic Z, Bresee JS, et al: Treatment of respiratory syncytial virus infection with vitamin A: a randomized, placebo-controlled trial in Santiago, Chile. *Pediatr Infect Dis J* 1996;15:782-786.

145. Laing I, Reidel F, Yap PL, et al: Atopy predisposing to acute bronchiolitis during an epidemic of respiratory syncytial virus. *Br Med J (Clin Res Ed)* 1982;284:1070-1072.

146. Nagayama Y, Sakurai N, Nakahara T, et al: Allergic predisposition among infants with bronchiolitis. *J Asthma* 1987;24:9-17.

147. Sims DG, Gardner PS, Weightman D, et al: Atopy does not predispose to RSV bronchiolitis or postbronchiolitic wheezing. *Br Med J (Clin Res Ed)* 1981;282:2086-2088.

148. Martinez FD, Morgan WJ, Wright AL, et al: Diminished lung function as a predisposing factor for wheezing respiratory illness in infants. *N Engl J Med* 1988;319:1112-1117.

149. Karron RA, Singleton RJ, Bulkow L, et al: Severe respiratory syncytial virus disease in Alaska native children. RSV Alaska Study Group. *J Infect Dis* 1999;180:41-49.

Chapter 5

Pathology and Pathogenicity

Caroline Breese Hall, MD

Professor of Pediatrics and Medicine
in Infectious Diseases,
University of Rochester Medical Center,
Rochester, New York

The prominent and piquant personality of RSV is illustrated by its ability to spread so effectively that essentially all humans experience infection within the first few years of life. Moreover, RSV may reinfect in subsequent years, sometimes within the same year. Thus, when RSV arrives in the community, it invariably finds a susceptible population, and one composed of all ages.

Modes of Inoculation and Infection

The singular contagiousness of RSV is not completely understood, but infection appears to require close contact with another person shedding RSV, or direct contact of infectious secretions on environmental surfaces.[1,2] Experiments on how nosocomial infections are spread have shown that medical personnel can become infected with RSV by large-particle aerosols or by touching surfaces contaminated with secretions and then touching their eyes or nasal mucosa.[1] However, persons who were exposed to infected infants at a distance greater than 6 feet did not become infected, suggesting that small-particle aerosol is an infrequent mode of transmission of RSV.

Although RSV is considered to be a labile virus, encased within infectious secretions, it may remain infectious on nonporous surfaces, such as countertops, for many hours.[2]

The eyes and nose are the major routes of inoculation, whether by aerosol or self-inoculation. The incubation period has been reported as varying between 2 and 8 days, but most likely averages 4 to 6 days. Viral replication then begins within the respiratory epithelium, with spread occurring mainly through intracytoplasmic ridges between epithelial cells. In infants and young children, spread of the virus commonly involves all levels of the conducting airways.

Histopathology and Pathogenesis of Clinical Signs

The characteristic histopathology in bronchiolitis is a lymphocytic peribronchiolar infiltration of the walls and surrounding tissue, with some edema.[3,4] Progression of infection is associated with the characteristic proliferation and necrosis of the bronchiolar epithelium. The sloughed necrotic epithelium and the increased mucus production result in obstruction of the infant's small airways. Air movement is impeded during both inspiration and expiration, but is more pronounced during expiration, as the lumen is narrowed further by the positive expiratory pressure. Clinically, this results in the characteristic wheezing heard during the infant's expiration. Many infants also demonstrate hyperinflation that results from the trapping of the air peripheral to the sites of partial occlusion of the small airways. Obstruction of airflow may become complete, leading to trapped air that eventually becomes absorbed. On chest x-ray, these multiple areas of atelectasis may sometimes, but not always, be visible. Atelectasis is more likely to develop in young infants because they have not yet developed fully the collateral channels that maintain alveolar expansion in the presence of airway obstruction. Measurement of

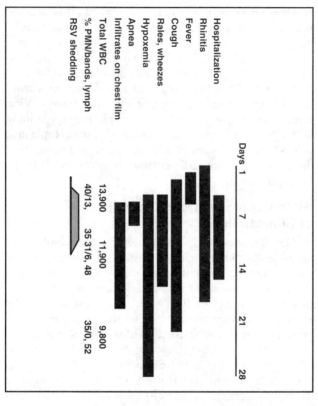

Figure 1: The course of this 8-week-old infant with pneumonia caused by RSV is characteristic of the course of young infants hospitalized with RSV lower respiratory tract disease. WBC = total white blood cell count per mm; % PMN/ bands, lymphs = percentage of polymorphonuclear cells, bands, and lymphocytes in the peripheral white blood cell count. (Reprinted with permission from Hall CB: Respiratory syncytial virus. In: Feigen RD, Cherry JD, eds. Textbook of Pediatric Infectious Diseases, 4th ed. Philadelphia, WB Saunders Co, 1998, pp 2084-2111.[6]

lung function during bronchiolitis shows an increase in lung volume and expiratory resistance.[5]

The predominant pathologic findings in pneumonia are an interstitial infiltration of mononuclear cells with surrounding edema and areas of necrosis, which lead to alveolar filling. Infants with lower respiratory tract disease may often clinically appear to have bronchiolitis or pneumonia, but in fact, have pathologic evidence of both. Some infants may have predominant signs of pneumonia at some times and at other times, those of bronchiolitis.

Restoration to normal of the histopathologic findings of RSV lower respiratory tract disease may lag behind the clinical signs of recovery. Histologically, recovery usually begins within the first week of illness, marked by the beginning regeneration of the epithelium of the bronchioles. Complete recovery, however, may take much longer. Ciliated cells may not reappear for weeks, and some morphologic alterations may persist even longer.

The histopathology of an infant with RSV infection shows in the small airways (75 μm to 300 μm) the characteristic findings of bronchiolitis: peribronchiolar infiltration of lymphocytes and edema of the bronchiolar walls and surrounding tissue. The lumen of the bronchioles are plugged with the sloughed, necrotic material.

Clinical Manifestations

The signs and symptoms from RSV infection can surprisingly vary not only among different infants, but even within hours in those with primary infection. The physiologic and clinical manifestations from the pathologic changes are best demonstrated in infants acquiring infection for the first time. Nevertheless, not all infants developing lower respiratory tract disease with a primary infection will develop the classical auscultatory changes and hyperinflation.

Although primary RSV infection in young infants may involve only the upper respiratory tract, the risk of subsequent spread to the lower respiratory tract is high. Estimates of primary infections involving the lower respiratory tract have been reported as ranging from 30% to 70%.[7-10] These estimates, however, are based on the presence of clinical chest findings and, sometimes, x-ray evidence of lower respiratory tract disease. Some infants with lower respiratory tract disease, nevertheless, may have little or no auscultatory manifestations and yet have diminishment in their arterial oxygen saturation levels, indicating the diffuse presence of RSV infection in the lower respiratory tract.

Infants with primary infection from RSV initially are most likely to have upper respiratory tract signs for 2 to 3 days before involvement of the lower respiratory tract. Mild nasal congestion and fever are common during this period. The fever is usually low grade and commonly disappears by the time of hospitalization or the development of clinical lower respiratory tract disease. As shown in Table 1, one third to one half of infants at the time of hospitalization are afebrile, indicating that fever may not be used as a reliable marker of severity of illness. Cough subsequently occurs and may become a major sign (Figure 1). It is frequently described as 'croupy' and may be paroxysmal, but it is not accompanied by a 'whoop' characteristic of pertussis. Although uncommon, hoarseness may occur.

Manifestations of lower respiratory tract disease are a deepening cough, an increased respiratory rate, and, sometimes, dyspnea with intercostal retractions of the chest muscles. The respiratory rate tends to be more rapid in bronchiolitis than in pneumonia, and expiration tends to be prolonged. The presence of intercostal retractions suggests that obstruction of the lower airway is both inspiratory and expiratory. Wheezing and hyperinflation are the most characteristic findings of bronchiolitis, but crackles may be heard in both bronchiolitis and pneumonia.

Table 1: Signs in Children With Respiratory Syncytial Viral Infection

	Percentage of Hospitalized Infants*	Percentage of Ambulatory Infants and Young Children**
Fever	45-65	74-100
Cough	97-100	83-100
Rhinitis	56-82	45-73
Pharyngitis	45-54	20-30
Hoarseness	—	6-20
Dyspnea	50-78	70-90
Retractions	36-68	40-100
Cyanosis	11-25	—
Wheezing	45-76	17-34
Rales	27-72	60-75
Rhonchi	59-78	15-90
Otitis	31	10-34
Conjunctivitis	9	15-30
Vomiting	45-52	20-27

Reprinted with permission from Hall CB: Respiratory syncytial virus. In: Feigen RD, Cherry JD, eds. *Textbook of Pediatric Infectious Diseases*, 4th ed. Philadelphia, WB Saunders Co, 1998, pp 2084-2111.[6]

* Data from Berglund[11] (93% of infants had lower respiratory tract disease), Gardner[12] (87% of infants had lower respiratory tract disease), and Hall CB (unpublished data on 637 hospitalized infants with lower respiratory tract disease).

** Data from Tyrell[13] (outpatients with bronchiolitis and pneumonia), Reilly[14] (patients from a British practice survey, two thirds with lower respiratory tract disease), and Hall CB (unpublished data on 434 outpatient children, one third with lower respiratory tract disease).

X-ray examination of the chest most frequently demonstrates multiple areas of interstitial infiltration and hyperinflation of the lung.[15-19] Hyperaeration is especially indicative of RSV infection and has been reported to occur in more than half of children hospitalized with RSV lower respiratory tract disease. Peribronchial thickening commonly accompanies the hyperaeration, but in 15% of patients, hyperaeration was the sole abnormality. Infiltrates in RSV lower respiratory tract disease may vary considerably and, in 20% to 25% of children, may appear as consolidated areas resulting from multiple areas of atelectasis. They are often located subsegmentally and often in the right upper or right middle lobe. The presence of pleural fluid has been reported in RSV lower respiratory tract disease but is so rare that it would generally indicate against the diagnosis of RSV infection.[15] The characteristic signs of hyperinflation and right or upper middle lobe atelectasis are not specific enough findings to allow differentiation from other respiratory viruses affecting the lower respiratory tract at this age, such as the parainfluenza and influenza viruses. Diminished arterial oxygen saturation levels are common, but are rarely associated with cyanosis.[20,21]

Most infants with lower respiratory tract disease begin to improve clinically within 3 to 4 days, although some degree of hypoxemia can remain, and the findings on chest x-ray are often present weeks after clinical recovery (Figure 1). Most children recover within a week, but commonly, the nasal congestion and especially the cough may continue for 1 to 3 weeks. In young infants, viral shedding can also be prolonged, lasting as long as 3 weeks.[22]

Primary infection may also be manifest as tracheobronchitis or as an upper respiratory tract infection with nasal congestion and cough. Otitis media is frequently associated with RSV primary infections, with or without lower respiratory tract involvement.[23-27] RSV has been isolated from middle ear fluids as the sole pathogen, but also in association with a bacterial pathogen. In some cases, only a bacterial pathogen has been detected. However, recent studies using the polymerase chain reaction (PCR) demonstrate that RSV is present in 75% of the middle ear effusions of children with documented RSV infection.[24] Infection by RSV with a concomitant bacterial pathogen has recently been shown to be associated with a worse clinical outcome of otitis media, including a prolonged duration of effusion and greater risk of treatment failure with antibiotics.[24,25,27]

Recurrent Infections

Repeated encounters with RSV are extremely common. The speed with which RSV spreads among groups of children, whether in day-care, school, or on the pediatric wards, provides high risk of re-exposure to the virus with each outbreak.[9,10,28] Frequently, an older child experiencing reinfection introduces RSV into the home, infecting an infant sibling. In older children, repeated infections usually manifest as milder illness, involving just the upper respiratory tract. This may be a common coldlike illness with or without fever, which in preschool children is often complicated by otitis media. A large portion of children with reinfection, nevertheless, will have involvement of the lower respiratory tract, such as tracheobronchitis or recurrent wheezing. Some may even have pneumonia.[9,10]

The severity of the second infection with RSV can be similar to that of the initial infection, according to longitudinal studies of children in day-care in Chapel Hill.[10] The attack rate for initial infection in day-care children in the child's first year was 98%, and for the second and third year was 75% and 65%, respectively. The first infection in this group appeared to have little effect on diminishing the degree of illness associated with the second infection. Only with the third infection did severity lessen.

Adults in contact with young children have an equally high risk of exposure to RSV and subsequent infection. In families with young children, other members frequently acquire RSV infection.[28] During a single outbreak, 43% of adult family members have been shown to become infected with RSV. Most of the infections in older family members are manifest as an upper respiratory tract infection characterized by nasal congestion, sore throat, and cough. Fever and earache, nevertheless, can accompany the illness, but less frequently than in young children. The severity, however, of the coldlike illness observed with RSV infections is greater than that associated with many other agents of upper respiratory tract infections, and the prolonged infection may also lead to the complications of sinusitis.[28-30] In one family study, only 32% of the family members recovered from their RSV infection within 1 week, while 74% of those with upper respiratory tract illnesses from other agents had recovered.[28] In some of the RSV-infected family members, symptoms remained for several weeks. Furthermore, about half of these previously healthy adults missed work when infected with RSV.

The prolonged coughing frequently leads to the diagnosis of tracheobronchitis or bronchitis, and wheezing may develop in patients with hyperreactive airways. Even in young, healthy adults without a known tendency for wheezing, RSV may be associated with airway hyperreactivity.[31] In a study of young adults with naturally acquired symptomatic RSV infection, serial pulmonary function testing showed elevated total pulmonary resistance and hyperreactivity of the airway in all of those tested. With cholinergic stimulus, this was still demonstrated for 8 weeks after the onset of illness.[31] The pulmonary function abnormalities usually correlate with the time required for the restoration of normal epithelium from the destruction caused by the viral inflammation.

Elderly, institutionalized adults are at high risk for developing severe, sometimes fatal, RSV infection.[32-34] Recently, however, RSV infection has been recognized as a potential cause of morbidity in healthy adults who live in the community. A study in Ohio examining the etiology of adults with pneumonia acquired in the community indicated that RSV accounted for 4.4% of the cases.[35] Although the authors believe this to be underestimated, RSV was, nevertheless, 1 of the 4 most common pathogens identified, including bacterial agents. RSV was not suspected to be the cause of pneumonia in any of the patients.

The RSV pneumonia in these patients was often manifest on chest x-ray, but often with a picture that could be interpreted as a bacterial pneumonia. Consolidation was evident in 40% of the chest x-rays and was lobar in distribution in 35%. Han et al[36] recently estimated the burden of RSV infection in the elderly. They estimated that 2% to 9% of the 687,000 hospitalizations and 74,000 deaths reported to occur annually from pneumonia in older populations were caused by RSV. With the estimated cost of 1 hospitalization for pneumonia caused by RSV at $11,000, the financial burden imposed by RSV disease in the elderly was judged to be $150 million to $680 million each year.

RSV Infection in High-Risk Populations

Neonates are at high risk for severe or complicated RSV infection. By virtue of age alone, infants in the first 4 to 6 weeks of life are at increased risk of hospitalization and complicated disease.[37] The clinical manifestations of RSV infection during the neonatal period may, however, be variable and less characteristic of classic viral lower respiratory tract disease observed in older infants. In some neonates, upper respiratory tract signs may be few and the predominant initial manifestations are general malaise, poor feeding, and irritability.[38] In these neonates, RSV infection may also be accompanied by periodic breathing and by apnea. The consequences of mild or unrecognized RSV infection in premature infants in neonatal intensive care units may be severe, resulting in unexpected episodes of apnea, bradycardia, and ventilatory complications.

Patients With Underlying Conditions

A high proportion of children hospitalized with RSV infection have an underlying disease, especially cardiopulmonary conditions and congenital disorders.[39-44] Although fatal infections with RSV are uncommon, one quarter to two thirds of the fatal infections occur in patients with these underlying conditions.

The risk factor usually identified in infants hospitalized with RSV lower respiratory tract disease is premature gestation or low birth-weight. Severity appears to correlate inversely with these factors. The additional presence of chronic lung disease places the infant at singularly high risk for rehospitalization for RSV infection after discharge from the neonatal intensive care unit. For infants with more severe prematurity and cardiopulmonary disease, the increased risk of rehospitalization with RSV infection continues into the second and third years of life.[43-48] In these children, RSV infection frequently is manifest as acute exacerbations or worsening of lower respiratory tract disease that doesn't respond to increased medical therapy alone and may require hospitalization and mechanical ventilation. Particularly at risk are infants who have required oxygen therapy at home within 6 months of the RSV infection.

Premature infants and infants in the first few weeks of life are at increased risk of apnea complicating their RSV infections.[49-51] The risk of apnea is highest in infants who have not yet reached 44 weeks postconceptional age. Bruhn et al[49] reported that 20% of infants younger than 6 months hospitalized with RSV infection in Denver had apnea. In studies in Rochester, NY, apnea was frequently shown to be the first manifestation of RSV infection, often occurring before any sign of respiratory illness was recognized.[50,51] The subsequent prognosis of infants with apnea associated with RSV infection, nevertheless, is generally good. Recurrence of apnea, even with subsequent respiratory infections, is infrequent in infants without underlying conditions.[51]

Infants with congenital heart disease have also been shown to have an increased rate of complicated or fatal RSV infection.[41,42] The initial prospective study of infants with congenital heart disease hospitalized with RSV infection, conducted in the 1980s, showed a high mortality in infants with functional, uncorrected cardiac lesions.[42] However, infants who had pulmonary hypertension associated with congenital heart disease had the highest mortality (73%). Subsequent surgical and medical advances have markedly improved the prognosis of children with congenital heart disease acquiring RSV infection, as indicated by the more recent Canadian study, in which the mortality in children with pulmonary hypertension and congenital heart disease was 9.4%.[41]

Immunocompromised Patients

The importance of RSV as an opportunistic pathogen in immunocompromised patients is getting increased recognition. RSV causes more severe, sometimes fatal, disease in patients who are immunocompromised.[39,52] In infants with congenital immunodeficiency syndromes, especially those with severe combined immunodeficiency, RSV causes devastating, disseminated pneumonia, and frequently, death.[52] In children undergoing chemotherapy for malignancy, RSV may cause a variably severe respiratory illness, depending on the degree of immunosuppression. In fatal cases, histologic sections of the lung can show disseminated involvement of the bronchioles and alveoli with a multinucleated giant-cell pneumonia.[53,54] Recent regimens of chemotherapy may cause several clinical manifestations in children acquiring RSV infection, which appear similar to other opportunistic pathogens.[39] Involvement of the lower respiratory tract, usually a diffuse pneumonia, often occurs even in older children when lower respiratory tract disease usually occurs in normal children. Shedding of the virus is also more prolonged than in immunosuppressed children, even in those with mild degrees of suppression.[39,55]

The recent increase in the number and types of transplant patients has refocused RSV's role and clinical presentation in the compromised host.[56-61] Concurrently, RSV's role as a major nosocomial pathogen has been re-emphasized, as many of the infections within transplant units are acquired nosocomially. RSV is frequently introduced onto the unit unnoticed, brought by visitors or medical personnel with mild upper respiratory tract infections. During a community outbreak of RSV, multiple introductions of different strains of RSV can occur.[62,63] The spread of the virus is rapid in transplant and oncology units and may continue well beyond the period of the community outbreak.

Shedding of RSV from infected patients on these units also tends to be prolonged, sometimes intermittent, and not always correlated with the severity of clinical findings. Nevertheless, most infected patients in transplant units have disease that is severe and complicated. Patients with lung transplants are at the highest risk of acquiring severe RSV and other respiratory viral infections.[64] The disease associated with RSV infection, however, is more severe than that associated with other respiratory viruses, such as influenza and parainfluenza viruses. In bone marrow transplant recipients studied by Ljungman,[65] the mortality from RSV infection was 60%, while the mortality from parainfluenza virus and influenza virus was 20% and 17%, respectively.

Studies at the M.D. Anderson Cancer Center in Houston, Texas have delineated RSV's major role among the respiratory viruses as an opportunistic infection.[57,58] In the center's adult cancer patients with respiratory illness, studied over a 3-year period, a respiratory virus, excluding herpes simplex virus and cytomegalovirus, was identified in 27% to 33% of the illnesses. Of these, RSV was most frequently isolated, accounting for 31% of the infections, most judged to be acquired nosocomially. Even these figures may underestimate the frequency of RSV infections in these patients, because serologic diagnosis was not used, and more than 1 sample per patient culture was uncommonly obtained.

RSV infection is commonly missed, indeed not even suspected, in these patients because the clinical presentation may mimic infections from pathogens more commonly thought of as opportunistic in these populations. Furthermore, rapid antigen testing in adults is frequently negative and more invasive procedures, such as bronchoalveolar lavage (BAL), may be necessary to establish RSV as the etiologic agent. Initially, RSV infection may be manifest silently or as an upper respiratory tract infection. Progression to the lower respiratory tract, however, occurs commonly and is often associated with the courses of immunosuppressive therapy. A diffuse, interstitial pneumonitis is the most common manifestation of lower respiratory tract involvement, but sometimes, the x-ray will be of a lobar pneumonia occasionally associated with pleural effusions, suggesting a bacterial etiology. The reported mortality in transplant units has generally ranged anywhere from 20% to 100%.[56,58,65-67] Early recognition of the RSV infection with infection control procedures and therapy and/or prophylaxis are integral to controlling the spread and severity of RSV infection in these units.[58]

The manifestations of RSV infection in HIV patients also appear to vary with the degree of immunosuppression.[68-70] In young children with HIV infection, the presentation of RSV infection is frequently similar to that observed in normal children, except that respiratory tract involvement, usually pneumonia, may continue to occur at older ages. Bacterial superinfection, particularly with gram-negative organisms, is observed in children with RSV and is a major cause of mortality.[69] Viral shedding also tends to be more prolonged, sometimes for months.

Patients With Other Underlying Conditions

RSV also appears to have an increasing but poorly defined role in exacerbation of other chronic illnesses. RSV as an instigator of asthmatic exacerbations has perhaps received the most recent attention, although the pathogenesis remains unclear and controversial (see Chapters 4 and 6). Patients with cystic fibrosis are at particularly high risk for developing RSV infection and respiratory complications that exacerbate their disease.[41,71-74] In studies by Hiatt et al,[71] children with cystic fibrosis and matched controls were followed over several respiratory seasons. In both groups, the same number of respiratory illnesses were reported, but children with cystic fibrosis with documented RSV infection had more frequent involvement of the lower respiratory tract and more severe illnesses, illustrated by a rate of hospitalization of more than 40%. Prospective studies by Armstrong et al[72] have also shown an increased severity of exacerbations associated with RSV infection in cystic fibrosis patients.

Children with underlying neurologic diseases and nephrotic syndrome also experience worsening of their underlying condition when acquiring RSV infection.[75,76] Little information is available about the role of RSV infection in augmenting diseases associated with other underlying conditions.

Differential Diagnosis

The major consideration in the differential diagnosis of lower respiratory tract disease with RSV infection in infants is asthma or hyperreactivity of the airways. To initially differentiate the two is often not possible, and indeed, the two may be combined. The first episode of wheezing may be associated with RSV infection, but may occur in a child with an atopic diathesis, especially in children with a strong family history of atopy. As shown by McIntosh et al,[77] 42% of wheezing episodes are associated with a viral infection, particularly with RSV. Thus, even the identification of RSV during a wheezing episode will not determine whether the child has a single episode of bronchiolitis and/or is asthmatic.

Gastric esophageal reflux may also mimic bronchiolitis, as well as the wheezing associated with an atopic predisposition. An infant with gastric esophageal reflux may present with the same clinical findings as bronchiolitis: wheezing, hyperaeration, and, sometimes, infiltrates on chest x-ray. The episodes may also be recurrent. Aspiration of a foreign body may produce a similar picture of wheezing and respiratory distress. Other entities that occasionally may cause wheezing and should be considered in the differential diagnosis include congestive heart failure and cystic fibrosis.

The differential diagnosis of recurrent RSV infection occurring in older children and adults is broad, variable, and often dependent on the presence of underlying disease. Most recurrent infections are of the upper respiratory tract, bronchitis, or tracheobronchitis, which all have multiple infectious causes. In patients with underlying conditions, as mentioned previously, the RSV infection may be manifest as another exacerbation of the underlying disease, or in the case of immunocompromised patients, as a respiratory illness caused by opportunistic infections. Most important in determining the role of RSV in these multiple presentations is an awareness of the epidemiology of RSV and its presence in the community, along with a ready suspicion that, at such times, this contagious virus can infect almost anyone.

References

1.   Hall CB, Douglas RG Jr: Modes of transmission of respiratory syncytial virus. *J Pediatr* 1981:99:100-103.

2.   Hall CB, Douglas RG Jr, Geiman JM: Possible transmission by fomites of respiratory syncytial virus. *J Infect Pediatr Dis* 1980;141:98-102.

3. Gardner PS, Turk DC, Aherne WA, et al: Deaths associated with respiratory tract infection in childhood. *Br Med J* 1967;4:316-320.

4. Aherne W, Bird T, Court SD, et al: Pathological changes in virus infections of the lower respiratory tract in children. *J Clin Pathol* 1970;23:7-18.

5. Wohl M: Present capacity to evaluate pulmonary function relevant to bronchiolitis. *Pediatr Res* 1977;11:252-253.

6. Hall CB: Respiratory syncytial virus. In: Feigen RD, Cherry JD, eds. *Textbook of Pediatric Infectious Diseases*, 4th ed. Philadelphia, WB Saunders Co, 1998, vol 2, pp 2084-2111.

7. Parrott RH, Kim HW, Arrobio JO, et al: Epidemiology of respiratory syncytial virus infection in Washington, DC. II. Infection and disease with respect to age, immunologic status, race, and sex. *Am J Epidemiol* 1973;98:289-300.

8. Loda FA, Glezen WD, Clyde WA Jr: Respiratory disease in group day care. *Pediatrics* 1972;49:428-437.

9. Glezen WP, Taber LH, Frank AL, et al: Risk of primary infection and reinfection with respiratory syncytial virus. *Am J Dis Child* 1986;140:543-546.

10. Henderson FW, Collier AM, Clyde WA Jr, et al: Respiratory-syncytial-virus infections, reinfections and immunity. A prospective, longitudinal study in children. *N Engl J Med* 1979;300:530-534.

11. Berglund V: Studies on respiratory syncytial virus infection. *Acta Paediatr Scand* 1967;176:1-40.

12. Gardner PS: Respiratory syncytial virus infections. *Postgrad Med J* 1973;49:788-791.

13. Tyrell DA: Discovering and defining the etiology of acute respiratory disease. *Am Rev Respir Dis* 1963;88:77-84.

14. Reilly CM, Stokes J Jr, McClelland L, et al: Studies of acute respiratory illness caused by respiratory syncytial virus. III. Clinical and laboratory findings. *N Engl J Med* 1961;264:1176-1182.

15. Rice RP, Loda F: A roentgenographic analysis of respiratory syncytial virus pneumonia in infants. *Radiology* 1966;87:1021-1027.

16. Simpson W, Hacking PM, Court SD, et al: The radiological findings in respiratory syncytial virus infection in children. II. The

correlation of radiological categories with clinical and virological findings. *Pediatr Radiol* 1974;2:155-160.

17. Khamapirad T, Glezen WP: Clinical and radiographic assessment of acute lower respiratory tract disease in infants and children. *Semin Respir Infect* 1987;2:130-144.

18. Friis B, Eiken M, Hornsleth A, et al: Chest x-ray appearances in pneumonia and bronchiolitis. Correlation to virological diagnosis and secretory bacterial findings. *Acta Paediatr Scand* 1990;79:219-225.

19. Davies HD, Wang EE, Manson D, et al: Reliability of the chest radiograph in the diagnosis of lower respiratory infections in young children. *Pediatr Infect Dis J* 1996;15:600-604.

20. Hall CB, Hall WJ, Speers DM: Clinical and physiological manifestations of bronchiolitis and pneumonia. Outcome of respiratory syncytial virus. *Am J Dis Child* 1979;133:798-802.

21. Mulholland EK, Olinsky A, Shann FA: Clinical findings and severity of acute bronchiolitis. *Lancet* 1990;335:1259-1261.

22. Hall CB, Douglas RG Jr, Geiman JM: Respiratory syncytial virus infections in infants: quantitation and duration of shedding. *J Pediatr* 1976;89:11-15.

23. Chonmaitree T, Howie VM, Truant AL: Presence of respiratory viruses in middle ear fluids and nasal wash specimens from children with otitis media. *Pediatrics* 1986;77:698-702.

24. Chonmaitree T, Owen MJ, Patel JA, et al: Effect of viral respiratory tract infection on outcome of acute otitis media. *J Pediatr* 1992;120:856-862.

25. Okamoto Y, Kudo K, Shirotori K, et al: Detection of genomic sequences of respiratory syncytial virus in otitis media with effusion in children. *Ann Otol Rhinol Laryngol Suppl* 1992;157:7-10.

26. Andrade MA, Hoberman A, Glustein J, et al: Acute otitis media in children with bronchiolitis. *Pediatrics* 1998;101:617-619.

27. Arola M, Ziegler T, Ruuskanen O: Respiratory virus infection as a cause of prolonged symptoms in acute otitis media. *J Pediatr* 1990;116:697-701.

28. Hall CB, Geiman JM, Biggar R, et al: Respiratory syncytial virus infections within families. *N Engl J Med* 1976;294:414-419.

29. Arola M, Ruuskanen O, Ziegler T, et al: Clinical role of respiratory virus infection in acute otitis media. *Pediatrics* 1990;86:848-855.

30. Monto AS, Cavallaro JJ: The Tecumseh study of respiratory illness. II. Patterns of occurrence of infection with respiratory pathogens, 1965-1969. *Am J Epidemiol* 1971;94:280-289.

31. Hall WJ, Hall CB, Speers DM: Respiratory syncytial virus infections in adults: clinical, virologic, and serial pulmonary function studies. *Ann Intern Med* 1978;88:203-205.

32. Sorvillo FJ, Huie SF, Strassburg MA, et al: An outbreak of respiratory syncytial virus pneumonia in a nursing home for the elderly. *J Infect* 1984;9:252-256.

33. Falsey AR, Treanor JJ, Betts RF, et al: Viral respiratory infections in the institutionalized elderly: clinical and epidemiologic findings. *J Am Geriatr Soc* 1992;40:115-119.

34. Mathur U, Bentley DW, Hall CB: Concurrent respiratory syncytial virus and influenza A infections in the institutionalized elderly and chronically ill. *Ann Intern Med* 1980;93:49-52.

35. Dowell SF, Anderson LJ, Gary HE Jr, et al: Respiratory syncytial virus is an important cause of community-acquired lower respiratory infection among hospitalized adults. *J Infect Dis* 1996;174:456-462.

36. Han LL, Alexander JP, Anderson LJ: Respiratory syncytial virus pneumonia among the elderly: an assessment of disease burden. *J Infect Dis* 1999;179:25-30.

37. Hall CB: Respiratory syncytial virus: A continuing culprit and conundrum. *J Pediatr* 1999;135:2-7.

38. Hall CB, Kopelman AE, Douglas RG Jr, et al: Neonatal respiratory syncytial viral infection. *N Engl J Med* 1979;300:393-396.

39. Hall CB, Powell KR, MacDonald NE, et al: Respiratory syncytial viral infection in children with compromised immune function. *N Engl J Med* 1986;315:77-81.

40. McMillan JA, Tristram DA, Weiner LB, et al: Prediction of the duration of hospitalization in patients with respiratory syncytial virus: use of clinical parameters. *Pediatrics* 1988;81:22-26.

41. Navas L, Wang E, de Carvalho V, et al: Improved outcome of respiratory syncytial virus infection in a high-risk hospitalized population of Canadian children. Pediatric Investigators Collaborative Network on Infections in Canada. *J Pediatr* 1992;121:348-354.

42. MacDonald NE, Hall CB, Suffin SC, et al: Respiratory syncytial viral infection in infants with congenital heart disease. *N Engl J Med* 1982;307:397-400.

43. Cunningham CK, McMillan JA, Gross SJ: Rehospitalization for respiratory illness in infants of less than 32 weeks' gestation. *Pediatrics* 1991;88:527-532.

44. Groothuis JR, Guiterrez KM, Lauer BA: Respiratory syncytial virus infection in children with bronchopulmonary dysplasia. *Pediatrics* 1988;82:199-203.

45. Groothuis JR, Salbenblatt CK, Lauer BA: Severe respiratory syncytial virus infection in older children. *Am J Dis Child* 1990;144:346-348.

46. Meert K, Heidemann S, Abella B, et al: Does prematurity alter the course of respiratory syncytial virus infection? *Crit Care Med* 1990;18:1357-1359.

47. Tammela OK: First-year infections after initial hospitalization in low birth weight infants with and without bronchopulmonary dysplasia. *Scand J Infect Dis* 1992;24:515-524.

48. Stevens TP, Sinkin RA, Hall CB, et al: Respiratory syncytial virus and premature infants born at 32 weeks' gestation or earlier: hospitalization and economic implications of prophylaxis. *Arch Pediatr Adolesc Med* 2000;154:55-61.

49. Bruhn FW, Mokrohisky ST, McIntosh K: Apnea associated with respiratory syncytial virus infection in young infants. *J Pediatr* 1977;90:382-386.

50. Anas N, Boettrich C, Hall CB, et al: The association of apnea and respiratory syncytial virus infection in infants. *J Pediatr* 1982;101:65-68.

51. Church NR, Anas NG, Hall CB, et al: Respiratory syncytial virus-related apnea in infants. Demographics and outcome. *Am J Dis Child* 1984;138:247-250.

52. Gelfand EW, McCurdy D, Rao CP, et al: Ribavirin treatment of viral pneumonitis in severe combined immunodeficiency disease. *Lancet* 1983;2:732-733.

53. Delage G, Brochu P, Robillard L, et al: Giant cell pneumonia due to respiratory syncytial virus. Occurrence in severe combined immunodeficiency syndrome. *Arch Pathol Lab Med* 1984;108:623-625.

54.   Shedden WI, Emery JL: Immunofluorescent evidence of respiratory syncytial virus infection in cases of giant-cell bronchiolitis in children. *J Path Bact* 1965;89:343-347.

55.   Ogra PL, Patel J: Respiratory syncytial virus infection and the immunocompromised host. *Pediatr Infect Dis J* 1988;7:246-249.

56.   Bowden RA: Respiratory virus infection after marrow transplant: the Fred Hutchinson Cancer Research Center experience. *Am J Med* 1997;102:27-30.

57.   Couch RB, Englund JA, Whimbey E: Respiratory viral infections in immunocompetent and immunocompromised persons. *Am J Med* 1997;102:2-9.

58.   Whimbey E, Englund JA, Couch RB: Community respiratory virus infections in immunocompromised patients with cancer. *Am J Med* 1997;102:10-18.

59.   Englund JA, Anderson LJ, Rhame FS: Nosocomial transmission of respiratory syncytial virus in immunocompromised adults. *J Clin Microbiol* 1991;29:115-119.

60.   Englund J, Piedra PA, Whimbey E: Prevention and treatment of respiratory syncytial virus and parainfluenza viruses in immunocompromised patients. *Am J Med* 1997;102:61-70.

61.   Garcia R, Raad I, Avi-Said D, et al: Nosocomial respiratory syncytial virus infections: prevention and control in bone marrow transplant patients. *Infect Control Hosp Epidemiol* 1997;18:412-416.

62.   Storch GA, Anderson LJ, Park CS, et al: Antigenic and genomic diversity within group A respiratory syncytial virus. *J Infect Dis* 1991;163:858-861.

63.   Mazzulli T, Peret TC, McGeer A, et al: Molecular characterization of a nosocomial outbreak of human respiratory syncytial virus on an adult leukemia/lymphoma ward. *J Infect Dis* 1999;180:1686-1689.

64.   Wendt CH: Community respiratory viruses: organ transplant recipients. *Am J Med* 1997;102:31-36.

65.   Ljungman P: Respiratory virus infections in bone marrow transplant recipients: the European perspective. *Am J Med* 1997;102:44-47.

66.   Harrington RD, Hooton TM, Hackman RC, et al: An outbreak of respiratory syncytial virus in a bone marrow transplant center. *J Infect Dis* 1992;165:987-993.

67.   Whimbey E, Champlin RE, Couch RB, et al: Community respiratory virus infections among hospitalized adult bone marrow transplant recipients. *Clin Infect Dis* 1996;22:778-782.

68.   King JC Jr: Community respiratory viruses in individuals with human immunodeficiency virus infection. *Am J Med* 1997;103:19-24.

69.   Chandwani S, Borkowsky W, Krasinski K, et al: Respiratory syncytial virus infection in human immunodeficiency virus-infected children. *J Pediatr* 1990;117:251-254.

70.   Atkins J, Karimi P, Doyle M: RSV infection among HIV-exposed infants: is RSV-IVIG indicated. *Pediatr Res* 1998;43(4): 140A.

71.   Hiatt PW, Grace SC, Kozinetz CA, et al: Effects of viral lower respiratory tract infection on lung function in infants with cystic fibrosis. *Pediatrics* 1999;103:619-626.

72.   Armstrong D, Grimwood K, Carlin JB, et al: Severe viral respiratory infections in infants with cystic fibrosis. *Pediatr Pulmonol* 1998;26:371-379.

73.   Hordvik N, Konig P, Hamory B, et al: Effects of acute viral respiratory tract infections in patients with cystic fibrosis. *Pediatr Pulmonol* 1989;7:217-222.

74.   Abman SH, Ogle JW, Butler-Simon N, et al: Role of respiratory syncytial virus in early hospitalizations for respiratory distress of young infants with cystic fibrosis. *J Pediatr* 1988;113: 826-830.

75.   MacDonald NE, Wolfish N, McLaine P, et al: Role of respiratory viruses in exacerbations of primary nephrotic syndrome. *J Pediatr* 1986;108:378-382.

76.   Hall CB, Powell KR, Schnabel KC, et al: Risk of secondary bacterial infection in infants hospitalized with respiratory syncytial viral infections. *J Pediatr* 1988;113:266-271.

77.   McIntosh K, Ellis EF, Hoffman LS, et al: The association of viral and bacterial respiratory infections with exacerbation of wheezing in young asthmatic children. *J Pediatr* 1973;82:578-590.

Chapter 6

Immune Response

Robert C. Welliver, MD

Department of Pediatrics, Division of Infectious Diseases,
State University of New York at Buffalo
and Children's Hospital of Buffalo, New York

The possibility that the immune response to respiratory syncytial virus (RSV) infection can provide partial immunity to illness while also contributing to the pathogenesis of lower respiratory disease has fascinated investigators for decades. The most severe expression of illness is observed in infants, who generally have substantial, transplacentally acquired titers of neutralizing antibody. Clinicians have recently demonstrated that RSV is a common cause of pneumonia and wheezing in the elderly, despite a lifetime of repeated RSV infections. The same paradox holds for cell-mediated immune responses to the virus. Adequate T-cell responses are required for termination of viral replication and perhaps for restriction of the virus to the upper respiratory tract. In contrast, evidence suggests that exaggerated cell-mediated immune responsiveness to some viral antigens can provoke unusually severe forms of respiratory illness.

This chapter describes how the immune response to RSV is initiated and sustained. Ways in which the various components of the immune response contribute to protection against infection or, alternatively, contribute to disease pathogenesis, are also reviewed.

Initiation of Inflammatory Responses to Viral Agents

The inflammatory response to RSV infection is probably initiated by infected epithelial cells. Infection of monolayers of epithelial cells with RSV, rhinoviruses, and other viruses causes the activation of the transcription factors activator protein-1, nuclear factor (NF)-B, NF-IL6 and C/EBP.[1,2] This, in turn, results in the release of numerous proinflammatory cytokines and chemokines, including interleukins (IL)1, 6, 8, and 11; granulocyte-macrophage colony-stimulating factor (GM-CSF); tumor necrosis factor alpha (TNFα); the chemokines known as regulated upon activation, normal T-cell expressed and secreted (RANTES); and macrophage inflammatory protein-1 alpha (MIP-1α).[3-6] Many of these cytokines induce the expression of intercellular adhesion molecule (ICAM)-1 and class 1 major histocompatibility complex (MHC) antigens on human nasal and airway epithelial cells in culture.[2,7,8] Increased expression of these structures may ease recognition of infected cells by lymphocytes and supply a mechanism for inflammatory cells to adhere to the infected epithelium.

ICAM-1 expression may also be a critical step in asthma induction. The expression of ICAM-1 is quantitatively greater on bronchial epithelial cells obtained from allergic asthmatics in comparison to normal controls or patients with chronic bronchitis. The degree of ICAM-1 expression correlates with the severity of asthma symptoms.[9] In addition, in a primate model of asthma, administration of monoclonal antibodies to ICAM-1 reduced both airway eosinophilia and bronchial hyperreactivity.[10] Therefore, induction of ICAM-1 may be important in establishing the inflammatory response in both allergic asthma and in virus-induced wheezing. Table 1 summarizes the features of the immune response seen after both viral infections and allergic asthma.

Table 1: Common Features of Immune Responses in Virus-Induced Wheezing and Allergic Asthma

Feature	Viral Infections	Asthma
Transcription factors activated	Activator protein-1, NFκB, NF-IL6	Same factors presumed to be activated
Epithelial cell chemokines and cytokines	IL1β, IL6, IL8, IL11	IL1, IL6, IL8
	GM-CSF, TNFα	Same
	MCP1-4, RANTES, MIP1α, eotaxin	Same
Epithelial cell activation markers	ICAM-1, MHC-1	ICAM-1, HLA-DR
Predominant bronchoalveolar cell type	Neutrophils	Macrophages

Feature	Viral Infections	Asthma
Cells in mucosal biopsies or lung parenchyma tissue	Lymphocytes (CD4+ & CD8+)	CD4+ lymphocytes, lsome CD8+
	Eosinophils with recurrent wheezing episodes	Eosinophils most prevalent α cell type
Cytokines	IFNγ, some IL4, minimal IL5	IL4, IL5, some IFNγ
Specific IgE responses	RSV, parainfluenza virus, *C pneumoniae*	Allergens
Mediators of airway obstruction	Histamine, tryptase, cysteinyl leukotrienes, kinins, prostaglandins, eosinophil cationic protein	Same, also eosinophil major basic protein
Nitric oxide (exhaled)	Increased with recurrent wheezing	Increased in asthma

See text for references

Generation of Chemokines

Chemokines are chemotactic cytokines that attract leukocytes to inflammation sites. More than 40 chemokines have been identified; they are structurally similar, sharing amino acid sequence homology ranging from 20% to 70%.[11] Interleukins (IL) 6 and 8 have chemotactic activity for most types of leukocytes. Epithelial cells infected with RSV, influenza, or rhinoviruses release these chemokines.[3,12,13] In addition, IL6 and IL8, as well as tumor necrosis factor-α, IL1-β, and GM-CSF have been detected in respiratory secretions of children with viral upper respiratory infections (URI),[14] with virus-induced wheezing,[15] and with allergic asthma.[16-18] An important role for these mediators in asthma development has, therefore, been suggested. However, these chemokines are also released in response to several bacterial and noninfectious insults to the airway, in which wheezing does not occur. Other chemokines are somewhat more selective in their chemotactic activity for eosinophils, basophils, and T-lymphocytes, the cells that infiltrate the airway in asthma. These include RANTES, macrophage inflammatory protein-1α, and 1-β (MIP-1α and MIP-1β), the monocyte chemotactic proteins (MCP), and eotaxin. These chemokines are found in increased concentrations in bronchoalveolar lavage (BAL) fluids from asthmatics.[17] The quantities of RANTES and MCP-1 in BAL correlate with lymphocyte counts in the same fluids. In addition, the eosinophil chemotactic activity of BAL fluids is blocked by preincubation of fluids with antibodies to RANTES and MCP-3, indicating a functional role for these compounds in attracting eosinophils to the airway. Intranasal endobronchial challenge with allergens causes the release of these chemokines at the challenge site.[18,19] Finally, intranasal administration of RANTES to allergic subjects incites an inflammatory response consisting of eosinophils, basophils, and lymphocytes, but not monocytes, neutrophils, or epithelial cells.[20] Therefore, clinicians assume these compounds may play a more specific role in creating the characteristic inflammation observed in asthma.

These compounds are also released by epithelial cells infected with RSV. By using molecular biologic techniques and enzyme-linked immunosorbent assay (ELISA), clinicians have documented the release of RANTES from cultures of epithelial cells obtained from nasal epithelial biopsies and adenoidal tissue, from cell cultures of tracheal (HEP-2), large bronchial and small airway (SAE) epithelial cells, and from type II pneumocytes (A549) all after infection with RSV and influenza virus.[21-24] In one study, RSV infection increased expression of RANTES, but not IL8, growth-related peptide-α or MCP-1.[21] One study demonstrated a greater release of RANTES from lower airway epithelial cells infected with RSV than those from the upper airway.[22] In the study, MCP-1 and MIP-1 were produced by small airway and alveolar cells, but not by bronchial epithelial cells. Another study reported that eotaxin is released by RSV-infected type II pneumocytes.[25] Therefore, it appears that release of these chemokines by airway epithelial cells is greatest in the terminal airways, the site where inflammation and airway obstruction caused by RSV infection are also the most severe.

In in vivo studies, the presence of IL8, RANTES, and MIP-1α have been evaluated both in infants with RSV bronchiolitis and in older children with virus-induced exacerbations of asthma caused by a variety of viral agents.[26-28] In comparison to healthy controls, concentrations of all 3 compounds were increased in secretions during acute wheezing. Quantities of these compounds correlated with the number of inflammatory cells in respiratory tract secretions, suggesting that these compounds may be important in initiating the inflammatory response to RSV infection. Perhaps more importantly, concentrations of MIP-1α, but not other chemokines, were highly correlated with the quantity of eosinophil cationic protein in tracheal secretions of infants with severe RSV bronchiolitis.[29] MIP-1α may, therefore, be important in inducing the migration and degranulation of eosinophils in the airway during RSV infection.

Preliminary studies[30] from our laboratory evaluated the release of RANTES, MIP-1α, and eotaxin into the airway during acute RSV infection. We found that all 3 chemokines were released during RSV infection. However, the quantities of RANTES and of eotaxin were similar in infants with wheezing and with URI caused by RSV infection. In contrast, MIP-1α was found in greater quantities in infants with wheezing than in those with URI alone. Quantities of MIP-1α and eotaxin, but not RANTES, were directly related to the degree of hypoxia. The results of these in vitro and in vivo studies suggest that the chemokines relevant to the pathogenesis of bronchiolitis are similar to those released in allergic asthma, and that MIP-1α might be of particular importance in the pathogenesis of virus-induced wheezing.

Inflammatory Cells Infiltrating the Lung

Neutrophils and macrophages. Neutrophils are the predominant cells found in BAL fluids taken from infants with bronchiolitis[31] and are also the cell type most frequently identified in nasal secretions of patients with rhinovirus URI.[32] Peripheral blood neutrophils (obtained from healthy adult volunteers) damage RSV-infected monolayers of epithelial cells in vitro.[33,34] Normal neutrophils incubated with RSV also release IL8, MIP-1α, and MIP-1β, and myeloperoxidase.[35] Therefore, neutrophils could augment inflammatory responses during RSV infection, although the activity of cells recovered directly from the airway has not been evaluated.

The role of macrophages in RSV-induced wheezing is also uncertain. RSV can infect macrophages to a limited extent. Once infected, macrophages briefly secrete IL12 and IFNγ, and release IL6, IL8, and TNFα over longer periods.[36,37] Thus, macrophages can also contribute to the earliest immune response to RSV infection.

In summary, neutrophils and macrophages can participate in the initiation of the inflammatory response to RSV infection. It is conceivable that these cells damage infected airway epithelial cells, and might even contribute to the sloughing of the epithelium which occurs in bronchiolitis. On the other hand, neutrophils and macrophages are also the most common cell type observed in bacterial pneumonia and a variety of other insults to the airway in which wheezing does not occur. Therefore, while further investigation is warranted, it is difficult to attribute an important role to these cells in the pathogenesis of allergic or virus-induced obstructive airway disease.

Lymphocytes. As noted above, neutrophils make up 80% to 90% of inflammatory cells present in BAL fluids of infants with RSV bronchiolitis.[31] In contrast, lymphocytes comprise the majority of cells seen in lung tissue obtained at autopsy of infants with bronchiolitis; neutrophils are observed infrequently.[38,39]

Most lymphocytes in BAL fluids of infants with RSV bronchiolitis are CD4+, similar to BAL lymphocytes observed in asthmatics.[31] This is surprising, since one might expect that most responding cells during viral infections would be CD8+ cytotoxic lymphocytes. No information is available on the subsets of T-lymphocytes present in the lung in bronchiolitis. CD4+ cells predominate in peripheral blood during acute bronchiolitis, while CD8+ cells are more common in other viral infections not associated with wheezing.[40,41] Rhinovirus infections result in modest lymphocytic infiltration of the lower airway, consisting of both CD4+ and CD8+ cells.[42] While more studies are needed before conclusions can be drawn, it nevertheless appears possible that both allergic and virus-induced wheezing can be mediated by aberrant CD4+ lymphocyte responses to allergens or viral antigens.

Eosinophils. Eosinophils are not detected in lung tissues of infants with fatal bronchiolitis,[38,39] even though they are present in normal lung tissues of infants of the same age. Eosinophil cationic protein (ECP), an inflammatory protein present in eosinophil granules, is found in high concentrations in nasopharyngeal secretions of infants with RSV bronchiolitis.[43,44] These findings suggest that airway eosinophils degranulate at RSV infection. The results of these[43,44] and 2 subsequent studies also suggest that this degranulation occurs to a greater degree in infants with wheezing caused by RSV and other viruses in comparison with infants with simple viral URI alone.[45,46] With RSV infection, eosinophils may not be evident in the airway in infancy because RSV infection suppresses eosinophilia in most, but not all, infants.[45]

In contrast to RSV, infections with rhinovirus induce airway eosinophilia in most infected patients, although the response is more persistent in asthmatic individuals.[42] An asthmatic infant with fatal rhinovirus-induced wheezing had numerous eosinophils in lung tissue at autopsy.[47] These differences in the appearance of eosinophils in the lung may be more a function of the host's age or atopic status rather than the infecting virus.

Recently, in a finding of great potential significance, the quantity of ECP released at the time of bronchiolitis predicted the rate of recurrent wheezing in the first year after bronchiolitis in 2 out of 3 studies.[48-50] Martinez et al[51] found that most infants manifested a reduction in eosinophil counts in their first episode of lower respiratory illness (pneumonia, croup, or wheezing). However, infants who maintained their eosinophil counts with these illnesses were more likely to have physician-diagnosed asthma at age 6. We have completed a study of infants with RSV bronchiolitis followed through age 7.[52] Infants who had detectable eosinophils in their peripheral blood at the time of RSV bronchiolitis were more likely to have asthma at age 7 than infants with suppressed eosinophil counts during bronchiolitis. Therefore, eosinophilia (and eosinophil degranulation) with bronchiolitis can predict recurrent wheezing and childhood asthma. This suggests that an immunologic process associated with eosinophilia and contributing to airway obstruction is common to both bronchiolitis in infancy and childhood asthma. Therefore, the link between bronchiolitis and subsequent asthma may not be a causative relationship, but instead may be a reflection of an immunologic anomaly common to both conditions. The nature of this anomaly is uncertain, but is under investigation. A proposed scheme by which the immune response to viral infections might result in airway obstruction is illustrated in Figure 1.

Functional Responses

Antibody formation. Antibody responses to RSV in the IgM, IgG, and IgA isotypes occur in both serum and respiratory secretions after RSV infection.[53-56] Responses are somewhat diminished in infants aged less than 6 months than in older infants. This reduced antibody responsiveness in younger infants may be caused by the inhibitory effects of transplacentally acquired maternal antibody in serum, or may reflect immunologic immaturity in the infant. Second infections occurring in the same infant are associated with enhanced serum and secretory antibody responses in all 3 isotypes.[53,54] Antibody titers are more easily measured by immunofluorescence or ELISA assays than by the more time-consuming neutralization assay, but titers measured by these methods correlate well with each other.[56]

Primary RSV infections occur frequently in infants despite maternally acquired antibody in the serum of the infant.[57] Reinfections with the virus occur throughout life, despite high titers of neutralizing antibody acquired in previous infection.[58] How RSV is able to escape neutralization and infect the host in the face of pre-existing antibody remains unknown. Nevertheless, both the quantity of virus

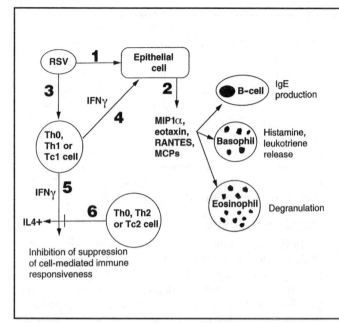

Figure 1: *Proposed mechanism by which respiratory syncytial virus (RSV) and other viruses may induce airway obstruction following infection.*

shed and the severity of illness are reduced with succeeding infections in healthy children. This partial protection is correlated better with the titer of antibody in serum, rather than that in respiratory secretions.[58] The overall beneficial effect of pre-existing serum antibody in RSV infection has been demonstrated by passive immunization studies in infants at high risk for severe RSV disease.[59-61] In these studies, the monthly administration of either polyclonal human antibody against the fusion protein of RSV or humanized mouse monoclonal antibody against the fusion protein each resulted in approximately a 50% reduction in the need for hospitalization at subsequent RSV infection. Clinicians be-

Step 1. RSV infects epithelial cells, inducing the release of chemokines, such as macrophage inflammatory protein-1 α (MIP-1α), eotaxin, regulated on activation, normal T cell expressed and secreted (RANTES), and the monocyte chemotactic proteins (MCPs).

Step 2. These chemokines, in turn, attract and activate B-lymphocytes (stimulating IgE production), basophils (stimulating release of histamine and leukotrienes), and eosinophils (causing degranulation and release of other cytokines and mediators).

Step 3. RSV infection results in the activation of the human equivalent of T-helper type 1 (Th1) lymphocytes or perhaps type 1 cytotoxic lymphocytes, inducing the release of interferon gamma (IFNγ).

Step 4. IFNγ enhances the release of chemokines from RSV-infected epithelial cells.

Step 5. IFNγ inhibits the release of interleukin (IL) 4 from the human equivalent of T-helper type 2 (Th2) lymphocytes or perhaps type 2 cytotoxic lymphocytes.

Step 6. This, in turn, prevents the normal downregulation of cell-mediated responsiveness by IL4, permitting greater release of IFNγ and exacerbating the proposed pathway.

lieve the protective effect of antibody is caused by its neutralizing activity, although serum antibody is also capable of participating in antibody-dependent, cell-mediated cytotoxicity reactions.[62]

Several investigators[63-68] have demonstrated RSV-specific IgE responses in respiratory secretions and, to a lesser extent, in serum during RSV infection. Low titers of RSV-IgE are apparently generated in secretions of most infants with acute RSV infection,[63] but responses were greater in infants with bronchiolitis than in infants with URI alone in 2 studies.[64,65] In one study,[64] the magnitude of the IgE response correlated directly with the degree of hypoxia the infant experienced. Therefore, IgE-mediated hypersensitivity responses to RSV proteins can contribute to the pathogenesis of bronchiolitis.

Cell-mediated immune responses. RSV infection results in pneumonia more often in patients with deficiencies in T-lymphocyte number or function than in immunocompetent children.[69,70] In addition, viral shedding is prolonged in both immunocompromised patients, and patients receiving corticosteroids, suggesting that T-cells are important in terminating RSV infection and preventing the illness from spreading to the lower respiratory tract. However, clinicians have found it difficult to detect and study RSV-specific cytotoxic lymphocytes in infants with bronchiolitis,[71] so the protective effect of cytotoxic cells has not been established.

Evidence exists that lymphocytic hyperresponsiveness to viral antigens helps develop virus-induced wheezing. Infants who received a formalin-inactivated RSV vaccine developed in the 1960s exhibited striking lymphocyte reactivity to RSV antigen. The degree of lymphoproliferative activity to RSV antigen was much greater and more persistent than that induced by natural infection.[72] Enhanced airway obstruction occurred when these infants were subsequently infected with RSV.[73] These findings suggest that lymphocyte hypersensitization contributes to the severity of RSV bronchiolitis.

Similar to findings in recipients of the formalin-inactivated vaccine, clinicians later found that (nonimmunized) infants with RSV bronchiolitis develop evidence of cell-mediated immunity earlier in the illness than infants with RSV URI alone. Also, the persistence of heightened cell-mediated immunity can predict the frequency of recurrent wheezing after bronchiolitis.[74]

Induction of cytokines. IgE responses specific for RSV, parainfluenza viruses, and *Chlamydia pneumoniae* are associated with wheezing when patients are infected with each of these agents.[63-65,75,76] Rabatic et al[67] found increased expression of the low-affinity receptor for IgE (CD23) on B-lymphocytes from infants with acute RSV bronchiolitis in comparison with control infants and infants with

RSV-negative bronchiolitis. All patients with increased expression of CD23 had detectable RSV-IgE and IgG4 antibody responses. They concluded that RSV bronchiolitis was associated with upregulation of IgE synthesis. These data suggest that infection with RSV and other agents might be associated with the same type of T-helper type 2 (Th2) cytokine responses that can underlie the development of allergen-specific IgE antibody and eosinophil migration in allergic asthma.

To support this, Sigurs et al reported that infants with RSV bronchiolitis were more likely to have asthma (defined as wheezing at age 3) and more positive skin prick tests to allergens (but not more atopic eczema) than infants who did not have bronchiolitis.[77] Renzi et al studied infants 5 months after an episode of bronchiolitis, and found persistently elevated CD23 expression and evidence of continued lymphocyte activation.[78] Roman et al[79] found a reduced number of suppressor lymphocytes in infants with RSV bronchiolitis. These findings might lead to the conclusion that RSV infection uncovers an allergic diathesis featuring unregulated lymphocyte activity, eosinophilia, and increased IgE production, possibly to a variety of allergens. In this regard, some clinicians suggest that asthma development might result from no exposure in early life to infections that promote Th1 cytokine responses. These infants would then be unable to prevent the development of Th2 cytokine responses upon exposure to allergens, and, therefore, to prevent the development of atopy.[80]

These studies of Th2 responses to RSV infection are limited because they cannot determine whether the immunologic biases identified were induced by RSV infection or if they were already present, representing the inherent immunologic status of the host. In this regard, several studies demonstrate that infants of asthmatic or atopic parents have elevated IgE antibody titers in cord blood specimens, greater expression of CD23 antigen on

B-lymphocytes, and reduced IFNγ synthesis by peripheral blood mononuclear cells.[81,82] This suggests that the Th2-like responses observed during convalescence from RSV infection may predate, rather than be induced by, the infection.

If these immunologic features are induced by RSV infection, you would expect Th2 cytokines to predominate in wheezing, RSV-infected patients. We recently determined the quantities of IL4 and IFNγ in nasopharyngeal secretions of infants with RSV infection. Rather than a role for Th2 cytokines in virus-induced wheezing, we found higher concentrations of IFNγ in infants and children with bronchiolitis or recurrent wheezing caused by RSV, while IL4 was the predominant cytokine in patients with URI alone and in healthy control infants.[83] IFNγ was also found in greater quantities than IL4 in samples of serum obtained during acute RSV bronchiolitis in a separate study by Renzi et al.[78] Oymar et al found only low concentrations of IL5 in serum of infants with bronchiolitis and older children with virus-induced wheezing.[84] Thus, since IFNγ is the predominant cytokine secreted during RSV bronchiolitis (and IL4 and IL5 are not increased), the findings suggest that RSV infection does not induce a persistent Th2 bias in the host. The predominance of IL4 in secretions during RSV infection in infants with URI might suggest that the secretion of IL4 has some protective function, rather than the pathologic role proposed for this cytokine in asthma. IL4 downregulates cell-mediated immune responses. Therefore, it is possible to conceive of bronchiolitis (in which IFNγ becomes relatively more predominant) as being the result of an over-response of the cell-mediated immune system to RSV infection.

In some strains of mice vaccinated with the G protein of RSV, subsequent challenge with RSV is accompanied by the production of the Th2 cytokines, IL4 and IL5.[85,86] These mice develop an unusual pulmonary illness characterized by eosinophils infiltrating the airway. In contrast, mice vaccinated with the F protein predominantly induce the Th1 cytokine IFNγ, and no eosinophils infiltrate the lung upon subsequent RSV challenge of these mice. The relevance of these findings to human illness is uncertain, in that stimulation of mouse and human lymphocytes with intact, whole virus predominantly induces IFNγ, and little IL4 or IL5.[85-87]

We speculate that the pathogenesis of airway obstruction from RSV infection may be mediated by the numerous proinflammatory activities of IFNγ. These include the enhanced release of RANTES from RSV-infected epithelial cells in the presence of IFNγ,[22] the potentiation of TNFα and MIP-1α release by macrophages stimulated with IFNγ,[88] and the enhanced release of histamine[89] and leukotrienes[90] from basophils and eosinophils after incubation with IFNγ. RANTES and MIP-1α are capable of enhancing IgE synthesis induced by IL4 in human B-lymphocytes,[91] perhaps explaining why some infants with bronchiolitis can release excessive quantities of virus-specific IgE antibody even though IL4 concentrations remain at baseline levels.[64,83] Finally MIP-1α is a known activator of human basophils and mast cells[92] and may also direct the recruitment of CD4+ lymphocytes to the airway.[93]

Release of mediators or airway obstruction. RSV (and other infectious agents) can induce specific IgE antibody responses in respiratory secretions[63,64,75] and serum[65,76,77] during acute infection. Infants and children with virus-induced wheezing may also have detectable quantities of histamine,[64,94,95] tryptase,[96] prostaglandins,[95] and leukotrienes[83,97] in respiratory secretions and plasma during acute infection. RSV induces the expression of 5-lipoxygenase (a key enzyme in leukotriene synthesis) in human bronchial epithelial cells, and the release of small amounts of leukotrienes in supernatants of these cells.[98] Alveolar macrophages of wheezing infants exhibit enhanced release of thromboxanes and leukotriene B4.[99] Rhinoviruses generate production of kinins in nasal secretions.[32] Therefore, the mediators important in the pathogenesis of allergic asthma are also induced in virus-induced wheezing. In many cases, the amounts of these mediators in virus-induced wheezing are similar or slightly greater than those found in patients with URI caused by the same infectious agents. Therefore, the airways of children who develop wheezing may be more susceptible to the effects of these agents, just as adults with asthma may have airways that are more reactive to these compounds.[100]

These findings suggest that RSV frequently causes sufficient inflammatory airway response to cause obstruction and wheezing whether or not a subject is atopic. Infection with these viruses may also increase the reactivity of the airway to mediators released at the time of infection. In contrast, rhinoviruses do not appear capable of provoking enough inflammation to cause airway obstruction in normal people. However, rhinoviruses enhance several inflammatory processes (lymphocyte activation, eosinophil infiltration, and histamine release) already underway in asthmatics, which, therefore, may cause episodes of wheezing.

Nitric oxide release. Quantities of exhaled nitric oxide are increased in asthma, probably reflecting the degree of inflammation in the airway.[99] Nitric oxide may be an important component of the immune response to viral infections as well.[101] Nitric oxide inhibits the release of the proinflammatory cytokines IL6 and IL8 by epithelial cells infected with rhinoviruses.[102] In this study, viral replication was also inhibited by nitric oxide, so it remains uncertain whether there is a direct effect of nitric oxide on cytokine release.

Clinicians recently demonstrated that exhaled nitric oxide is also increased in children with recurrent wheezing, in comparison with healthy children.[103] Children with first episodes of wheezing had intermediate levels of exhaled nitric oxide, which did not differ significantly from those of healthy children. Children with URI without wheezing were not included, so clinicians could not determine if increases in exhaled nitric oxide are a result of inflammatory responses to viral infections in general, or bear a specific relationship to wheezing illnesses. Unfortunately, a preliminary study suggests that inhaled nitric oxide does not improve lung function in infants with severe RSV bronchiolitis.[104]

The Immune Response to RSV Infection and the Development of Childhood Asthma

The immune response to RSV and other viral infections is similar in many ways to allergen exposure. There are, no doubt, many features which are also common to the response to bacterial infections, during which wheezing does not occur. Nevertheless, airway infiltration with lymphocytes and eosinophils represents a clear-cut difference, and other differences may eventually be recognized. These unique features are clues to the identity of the key elements of the immune response that contribute to RSV-induced wheezing.

If the immune response to viruses and allergens is similar, it provides an explanation for the link between viral bronchiolitis in infancy and the later development of asthma. That is, people who develop similar responses to viruses and allergens are likely to develop wheezing when exposed to each agent. It is, therefore, not necessary to assume that RSV infections in infancy create long-term destructive airway changes to explain the link to asthma in childhood. The existing evidence suggests that viral infections do not induce Th2 type immunologic responses.

Nevertheless, some short-term effects of viral infections may exist that predispose to recurrent wheezing. Virus-specific IgE responses[64] and airway eosinophilia after rhinovirus infections[42] are more prolonged with personal or family history of recurrent wheezing. The release of histamine[64,95] and possibly chemokines continues after a single episode of virus-induced wheezing in childhood. Chemokines themselves may be responsible for these variations in immune responses, which have traditionally been ascribed to the effects of Th2-like cytokines. Exposure of the airway to another viral infection or to an allergen during this vulnerable period might be more likely to result in recurrent wheezing. As a corollary, more intensive anti-inflammatory therapy immediately after an episode of virus-induced wheezing might reduce the frequency of recurrent wheezing episodes during this interval.

References

1.   Mastronarde JG, Monick MM, Mukaida N, et al: Activator protein-1 is the preferred transcription factor for cooperative interaction with nuclear factor-κB in respiratory syncytial virus-induced interleukin-8 gene expression in airway epithelium. *J Infect Dis* 1998;177:1275-1281.

2.   Chini BA, Fiedler MA, Milligan L, et al: Essential roles of NF-κB and C/EBP in the regulaton of intercellular adhesion molecule-1 after respiratory syncytial virus infection of human respiratory epithelial cell cultures. *J Virol* 1998;72:1623-1626.

3.   Noah TL, Becker S: Respiratory syncytial virus-induced cytokine production by a human bronchial epithelial cell line. *Am J Physiol* 1993;265:L472-L478.

4.   Einarsson O, Geba GP, Zhu Z, et al: Interleukin-11: stimulation in vivo and in vitro by respiratory viruses and induction of airways hyperresponsiveness. *J Clin Invest* 1996;97:915-924.

5.   Thomas LH, Friedland JS, Sharland M, et al: Respiratory syncytial virus-induced RANTES production from human bronchial epithelial cells is dependent on nuclear factor-κB nuclear binding and is inhibited by adenovirus-mediated expression of inhibitor of κBα. *J Immunol* 1998;161:1007-1016.

6.   Patel JA, Kunimoto M, Sim TC, et al: Interleukin-1a mediates the enhanced expression of intercellular adhesion molecule-1 in pulmonary epithelial cells infected with respiratory syncytial virus. *Am J Respir Cell Mol Biol* 1995;123:602-609.

7.   Matsuzaki Z, Okamoto Y, Sarashina N, et al: Induction of intercellular adhesion molecule-1 in human nasal epithelial cells

during respiratory syncytial virus infection. *Immunology* 1996;88:565-568.

8. Garofalo R, Mei F, Espejo R, et al: Respiratory syncytial virus infection of human respiratory epithelial cells up-regulates class I MHC expression through the induction of IFN-β and IL-1α. *J Immunol* 1996;157:2506-2513.

9. Vignola AM, Campbell AM, Chanez P, et al: HLA-DR and ICAM-1 expression on bronchial epithelial cells in asthma and chronic bronchitis. *Am Rev Respir Dis* 1993;148:689-694.

10. Wegner CD, Gundel RH, Reilly P, et al: Intercellular adhesion molecule-1 (ICAM-1) in the pathogenesis of asthma. *Science* 1990;247:456-459.

11. Luster AD: Chemokines—chemotactic cytokines that mediate inflammation. *N Engl J Med* 1998;338:436-445.

12. Matsukura S, Kokubu F, Noda H, et al: Expression of IL-6, IL-8, and RANTES on human bronchial epithelial cells, NCI-H292, induced by influenza virus A. *J Allergy Clin Immunol* 1996;98:1080-1087.

13. Johnston SL, Papi A, Bates PJ, et al: Low grade rhinovirus infection induces a prolonged release of IL-8 in pulmonary epithelium. *J Immunol* 1998;160:6172-6181.

14. Noah TL, Henderson FW, Wortman IA, et al: Nasal cytokine production in viral acute upper respiratory infection of childhood. *J Infect Dis* 1995;171:584-592.

15. Neuzil KM, Graham BS: Cytokine release and innate immunity in respiratory syncytial virus infection. *Sem Virol* 1996;7:255-264.

16. Noah TL, Henderson FW, Henry MM, et al: Nasal lavage cytokines in normal, allergic, and asthmatic school-age children. *Am J Respir Crit Care Med* 1995;152:1290-1296.

17. Alam R, York J, Boyars M, et al: Increased MCP-1, RANTES, and MIP-1α in bronchoalveolar lavage fluid of allergic asthmatic patients. *Am J Respir Crit Care Med* 1996;153:1398-1404.

18. Sim TC, Reece LM, Hilsmeier KA, et al: Secretion of chemokines and other cytokines in allergen-induced nasal responses: inhibition by topical steroid treatment. *Am J Respir Crit Care Med* 1995;152:927-933.

19. Holgate ST, Bodey KS, Janezic A, et al: Release of RANTES, MIP-1α, and MCP-1 into asthmatic airways following endobron-

chial allergen challenge. *Am J Respir Crit Care Med* 1997;156: 1377-1383.

20.   Kuna P, Alam R, Ruta U, et al: RANTES induces nasal mucosal inflammation rich in eosinophils, basophils, and lymphocytes in vivo. *Am J Respir Crit Care Med* 1998;157:873-879.

21.   Saito T, Deskin RW, Casola A, et al: Respiratory syncytial virus induces selective production of the chemokine RANTES by upper airway epithelial cells. *J Infect Dis* 1997;175:497-504.

22.   Olszewska-Pazdrak B, Casola A, Saito T, et al: Cell-specific expression of RANTES, MCP-1 and MIP-1α by lower airway epithelial cells and eosinophils infected with respiratory syncytial virus. *J Virol* 1998;72:4756-4764.

23.   Noah TL, Wortman IA, Becker S: The effect of fluticasone propionate on respiratory syncytial virus-induced chemokine release by a human bronchial epithelial cell line. *Immunopharmacology* 1998;39:193-199.

24.   Matsukura S, Kokubu F, Kubo H, et al: Expression of RANTES by normal airway epithelial cells after influenza virus A infection. *Am J Respir Cell Mol Biol* 1998;18:255-264.

25.   Garofalo RP, Welliver RC, Ogra PL: Clinical aspects of bronchial reactivity and cell-virus interaction. In: Ogra PL, Mestecky J, Lamm ME, et al, eds. *Mucosal Immunology,* 2nd ed. San Diego, Academic Press, 1999, pp 1223-1238.

26.   Becker S, Reed W, Henderson FW, et al: RSV infection of human airway epithelial cells causes production of the β-chemokine RANTES. *Am J Physiol* 1997;272:L512-L520.

27.   Sheeran P, Jafri H, Carubelli C, et al: Elevated cytokine concentrations in the nasopharyngeal and tracheal secretions of children with respiratory syncytial virus disease. *Pediatr Infect Dis J* 1999;18:115-122.

28.   Teran LM, Seminario MC, Shute JK, et al: RANTES, macrophage-inhibitory protein 1α, and the eosinophil product major basic protein are released into upper respiratory secretions during virus-induced asthma exacerbations in children. *J Infect Dis* 1999;179:677-681.

29.   Harrison AM, Bonville CA, Rosenberg HF, et al: Respiratory syncytial virus-induced chemokine expression in the lower airways: eosinophil recruitment and degranulation. *Am J Respir Crit Care Med* 1999;159:1918-1924.

30. Welliver RC: Chemokines and cytokines in virus-induced wheezing. Collaborative Investigators' Symposium, American Academy of Allergy, Asthma, and Immunology Annual Meeting, Orlando, FL, March 3, 1999.

31. Everard ML, Swarbrick A, Wrightham M, et al: Analysis of cells obtained by bronchial lavage of infants with respiratory syncytial virus infection. *Arch Dis Child* 1994;71:428-432.

32. Naclerio RM, Proud D, Lichtenstein LM, et al: Kinins are generated during experimental rhinovirus colds. *J Infect Dis* 1988;157:133-142.

33. Kaul TN, Faden H, Baker R, et al: Virus-induced complement activation and neutrophil-mediated cytotoxicity against respiratory syncytial virus (RSV). *Clin Exp Immunol* 1984;56:501-508.

34. Wang SZ, Xu H, Wraith A, et al: Neutrophils induce damage to respiratory epithelial cells infected with respiratory syncytial virus. *Eur Respir J* 1998;12:612-618.

35. Jaovisidha P, Peeples ME, Brees AA, et al: Respiratory syncytial virus stimulates neutrophil degranulation and chemokine release. *J Immunol* 1999;163:2816-2820.

36. Tsutsumi H, Matsuda K, Sone S, et al: Respiratory syncytial virus-induced cytokine production by neonatal macrophages. *Clin Exp Immunol* 1996;106:442-446.

37. Arnold R, Konig B, Galatti H, et al: Cytokine (IL-8, IL-6, TNF-α) and soluble TNF receptor-I release from human peripheral blood mononuclear cells after respiratory syncytial virus infection. *Immunology* 1995;85:364-372.

38. Downham MA, Gardner PS, McQuillin J, et al: Role of respiratory viruses in childhood mortality. *Br Med J* 1975;1:235-239.

39. Neilson KA, Yunis EJ: Demonstration of respiratory syncytial virus in an autopsy series. *Pediatr Pathol* 1990;10:491-502.

40. De Weerd W, Twilhaar WN, Kimpen JL: T cell subset analysis in peripheral blood of children with RSV bronchiolitis. *Scand J Infect Dis* 1998;30:77-80.

41. Raes M, Peeters V, Alliet P, et al: Peripheral blood T and B lymphocyte subpopulations in infants with acute respiratory syncytial virus bronchiolitis. *Pediatr Allergy Immunol* 1997;8:97-102.

42. Fraenkel DJ, Bardin PG, Sanderson G, et al: Lower airways inflammation during rhinovirus colds in normal and in asthmatic subjects. *Am J Respir Crit Care Med* 1995;151:879-886.

43. Garofalo R, Kimpen JL, Welliver RC, et al: Eosinophil degranulation in the respiratory tract during naturally acquired respiratory syncytial virus infection. *J Pediatr* 1992;120:28-32.

44. Colocho Zelaya EA, Orvell C, Strannegard O: Eosinophil cationic protein in nasopharyngeal secretions and serum of infants infected with respiratory syncytial virus. *Pediatr Allergy Immunol* 1994;5:100-106.

45. Garofalo R, Dorris A, Ahlstedt S, et al: Peripheral blood eosinophil counts and eosinophil cationic protein content of respiratory secretions in bronchiolitis: relationship to severity of disease. *Pediatr Allergy Immunol* 1994;5:111-117.

46. Pizzichini MM, Pizzichini E, Efthimiadis A, et al: Asthma and natural colds. Inflammatory indices in induced sputum: a feasibility study. *Am J Respir Crit Care Med* 1998;158:1178-1184.

47. Las Heras J, Swanson VL: Sudden death of an infant with rhinovirus infection complicating bronchial asthma: a case report. *Pediatr Pathol* 1983;1:319-323.

48. Reijonen TM, Korppi M, Kuikka L, et al: Serum eosinophil cationic protein as a predictor of wheezing after bronchiolitis. *Pediatr Pulmonol* 1997;23:397-403.

49. Koller DY, Wojnarowski C, Herkner KR, et al: High levels of eosinophil cationic protein in wheezing infants predict the development of asthma. *J Allergy Clin Immunol* 1997;99:752-756.

50. Oymar K, Bjerknes R: Is serum eosinophil cationic protein in bronchiolitis a predictor of asthma? *Pediatr Allergy Immunol* 1998;9:204-207.

51. Martinez FD, Stern DA, Wright AL, et al: Differential immune responses to acute lower respiratory illness in early life and subsequent development of persistent wheezing and asthma. *J Allergy Clin Immunol* 1998;102:915-920.

52. Ehlenfield DR, Cameron K, Welliver RC: Eosinophilia at the time of respiratory syncytial virus bronchiolitis predicts childhood reactive airway disease. *Pediatrics* 2000;105:79-83.

53. Welliver RC, Kaul TN, Putnam TI, et al: The antibody response to primary and secondary infection with respiratory syncytial virus: kinetics of class-specific responses. *J Pediatr* 1980;96:808-813.

54. Kaul TN, Welliver RC, Wong DT, et al: Secretory antibody response to respiratory syncytial virus infection. *Am J Dis Child* 1981;135:1013-1016.

55. McIntosh K, Masters HB, Orr I, et al: The immunologic response to infection with respiratory syncytial virus in infants. *J Infect Dis* 1978;138:24-32.

56. Kaul TN, Welliver RC, Ogra PL: Comparison of fluorescent-antibody, neutralizing-antibody, and complement-enhanced neutralizing-antibody assays for detection of serum antibody to respiratory syncytial virus. *J Clin Microbiol* 1981;13:957-962.

57. Glezen WP, Paredes A, Allison JE, et al: Risk of respiratory syncytial virus infection for infants from low-income families in relationshp to age, sex, ethnic group, and maternal antibody level. *J Pediatr* 1981;98:708-715.

58. Hall CB, Walsh EE, Long CE, et al: Immunity to and frequency of reinfection with respiratory syncytial virus. *J Infect Dis* 1991;163:693-698.

59. Groothuis JR, Simoes EA, Levin MJ, et al: Prophylactic administration of respiratory syncytial virus immune globulin to high-risk infants and young children. *N Engl J Med* 1993;329:1524-1530.

60. The PREVENT Study Group: Reduction of respiratory syncytial virus hospitalization among premature infants and infants with bronchopulmonary dysplasia using respiratory syncytial virus immune globulin prophylaxis. *Pediatrics* 1997;99:93-99.

61. The IMpact-RSV Study Group: Palivizumab, a humanized respiratory syncytial virus monoclonal antibody, reduces hospitalization from respiratory syncytial virus infection in high-risk infants. *Pediatrics* 1998;102:531-537.

62. Kaul TN, Welliver RC, Ogra PL: Development of antibody-dependent cell-mediated cytotoxicity in the respiratory tract after natural infection with respiratory syncytial virus. *Infect Immun* 1982;37:492-498.

63. Welliver RC, Kaul TN, Ogra PL: The appearance of cell-bound IgE in respiratory-tract epithelium after respiratory-syncytial-virus infection. *N Engl J Med* 1980;303:1198-1202.

64. Welliver RC, Wong DT, Sun M, et al: The development of respiratory syncytial virus-specific IgE and the release of histamine in nasopharyngeal secretions after infection. *N Engl J Med* 1981;305:841-846.

65. Bui RH, Molinaro GA, Kettering JD, et al: Virus-specific IgE and IgG4 antibodies in serum of children infected with respiratory syncytial virus. *J Pediatr* 1987;110:87-90.

66. Russi JC, Delfraro A, Borthagaray MD, et al: Evaluation of immunoglobulin E-specific antibodies and viral antigens in nasopharyngeal secretions of children with respiratory syncytial virus infections. *J Clin Microbiol* 1993;31:819-823.

67. Rabatic S, Gagro A, Lokar-Kolbas R, et al: Increase in CD23+ B cells in infants with bronchiolitis is accompanied by appearance of IgE and IgG4 antibodies specific for respiratory syncytial virus. *J Infect Dis* 1997;175:32-37.

68. Aberle JH, Aberle SW, Dworzak MN, et al: Reduced interferon-γ expression in peripheral blood mononuclear cells of infants with severe respiratory syncytial virus disease. *Am J Respir Crit Care Med* 1999;160:1263-1268.

69. Hall CB, Powell KR, MacDonald NE, et al: Respiratory syncytial viral infection in children with compromised immune function. *N Engl J Med* 1986;315:77-81.

70. Fishaut M, Tubergen D, McIntosh K: Cellular response to respiratory viruses with particular reference to children with disorders of cell-mediated immunity. *J Pediatr* 1980;96:179-186.

71. Isaacs D, Bangham CR, McMichael AJ: Cell-mediated cytotoxic response to respiratory syncytial virus in infants with bronchiolitis. *Lancet* 1987;2:769-771.

72. Kim HW, Leikin SL, Arrobio J, et al: Cell-mediated immunity to respiratory syncytial virus induced by inactivated vaccine or by infection. *Pediatr Res* 1976;10:75-78.

73. Fulginiti VA, Eller JJ, Sieber OF, et al: Respiratory virus immunization. I. A field trial of two inactivated respiratory virus vaccines; an aqueous trivalent parainfluenza virus vaccine and an alum-precipitated respiratory syncytial virus vaccine. *Am J Epidemiol* 1969;89:435-448.

74. Welliver RC, Kaul A, Ogra PL: Cell-mediated immune response to respiratory syncytial virus infection: relationship to the development of reactive airway disease. *J Pediatr* 1979; 94:370-375.

75. Welliver RC, Wong DT, Sun M, et al: Parainfluenza virus bronchiolitis. Epidemiology and pathogenesis. *Am J Dis Child* 1986;140:34-40.

76. Emre U, Skolovskaya N, Roblin PM, et al: Detection of anti-*Chlamydia pneumoniae* IgE in children with reactive airway disease. *J Infect Dis* 1995;172:265-267.

77. Sigurs N, Bjarnason R, Sigurbergsson F, et al: Asthma and immunoglobulin E antibodies after respiratory syncytial virus bronchiolitis: a prospective cohort study with matched controls. *Pediatrics* 1995;95:500-505.

78. Renzi PM, Turgeon JP, Yang JP, et al: Cellular immunity is activated and a TH-2 response is associated with early wheezing in infants after bronchiolitis. *J Pediatr* 1997;130:584-593.

79. Roman M, Calhoun WJ, Hinton KL, et al: Respiratory syncytial virus infection in infants is associated with predominant Th-2-like response. *Am J Respir Crit Care Med* 1997;156:190-195.

80. Shirakawa T, Enomoto T, Shimazu SI, et al: The inverse association between tuberculin responses and atopic disorder. *Science* 1997;275:77-79.

81. Rinas U, Horneff G, Wahn V: Interferon-γ production by cord-blood mononuclear cells is reduced in newborns with a family history of atopic disease and is independent from cord blood IgE-levels. *Pediatr Allergy Immunol* 1993;4:60-64.

82. Koning H, Baert MR, Oranje AP, et al: Development of immune functions related to allergic mechanisms in young children. *Pediatr Res* 1996;40:363-375.

83. van Schaik SM, Tristram DA, Nagpal IS, et al: Increased production of IFN-γ and cysteinyl leukotrienes in virus-induced wheezing. *J Allergy Clin Immunol* 1999;103:630-636.

84. Oymar K, Elsayed S, Bjerknes R: Serum eosinophil cationic protein and interleukin-5 in children with bronchial asthma and acute bronchiolitis. *Pediatr Allergy Immunol* 1996;7:180-186.

85. Hancock GE, Speelman DJ, Heers K, et al: Generation of atypical pulmonary inflammatory responses in BALB/c mice after immunization with the native attachment (G) glycoprotein of respiratory syncytial virus. *J Virol* 1996;70:7783-7791.

86. Johnson TR, Graham BS: Secreted respiratory syncytial virus G glycoprotein induces interleukin-5 (IL-5), IL-13, and eosinophilia by an IL-4-independent mechanism. *J Virol* 1999;73:8485-8495.

87. Jackson M, Scott R: Different patterns of cytokine induction in cultures of respiratory syncytial (RS) virus-specific human TH

cell lines following stimulation with RS virus and RS virus proteins. *J Med Virol* 1996;49:161-169.

88. Dery RE, Bissonnette EY: IFN-γ potentiates the release of TNF-α and MIP-1α by alveolar macrophages during allergic reactions. *Am J Respir Cell Mol Biol* 1999;20:407-412.

89. Chonmaitree T, Lett-Brown MA, Tsong Y, et al: Role of interferon in leukocyte histamine release caused by common respiratory viruses. *J Infect Dis* 1988;157:127-132.

90. Saito H, Hayakawa T, Mita H, et al: Augmentation of leukotriene C4 production by γ-interferon in leukocytes challenged with an allergen. *Int Arch Allergy Appl Immunol* 1988;87:286-293.

91. Kimata H, Yoshida A, Ishioka C, et al: RANTES and macrophage inflammatory protein 1α selectively enhance immunoglobulin (IgE) and IgG4 production by human B cells. *J Exp Med* 1996; 183:2397-2402.

92. Alam R, Forsythe PA, Stafford S, et al: Macrophage inflammatory protein-1α activates basophils and mast cells. *J Exp Med* 1992;176:781-786.

93. Schall TJ, Bacon K, Camp RD, et al: Human macrophage inflammatory protein α (MIP-1α) and MIP-1β chemokines attract distinct populations of lymphocytes. *J Exp Med* 1993;177:1821-1825.

94. Counil FP, Lebel B, Segondy M, et al: Cells and mediators from pharyngeal secretions in infants with acute wheezing episodes. *Eur Respir J* 1997;10:2591-2595.

95. Skoner DP, Fireman P, Caliguri L, et al: Plasma elevations of histamine and a prostaglandin metabolite in acute bronchiolitis. *Am Rev Respir Dis* 1990;142:359-364.

96. Everard ML, Fox G, Walls AF, et al: Tryptase and IgE concentrations in the respiratory tract of infants with acute bronchiolitis. *Arch Dis Child* 1995;72:64-69.

97. Volovitz B, Welliver RC, De Castro G, et al: The release of leukotrienes in the respiratory tract during infection with respiratory syncytial virus; role in obstructive airway disease. *Pediatr Res* 1988;24:504-507.

98. Behera AK, Kumar M, Matsuse H, et al: Respiratory syncytial virus induces the expression of 5-lipoxygenase and endothelin-1 in bronchial epithelial cells. *Biochem Biophys Res Commun* 1998;251:704-709.

99.   Azevedo I, de Blic J, Scheinmann P, et al: Enhanced arachidonic acid metabolism in alveolar macrophages from wheezy infants. Modulation by dexamethasone. *Am J Respir Crit Care Med* 1995;152:1208-1214.

100. Adelroth E, Morris MM, Hargreave FE, et al: Airway responsiveness to leukotrienes C4 and D4 and to methacholine in patients with asthma and normal controls. *N Eng J Med* 1986;315:480-484.

101. Reiss CS, Komatsu T: Does nitric oxide play a critical role in viral infections? *J Virol* 1998;72:4547-4551.

102. Sanders SP, Siekierski ES, Porter JD, et al: Nitric oxide inhibits rhinovirus-induced cytokine production and viral replication in a human respiratory epithelial cell line. *J Virol* 1998;72:934-942.

103. Baraldi E, Dario C, Ongaro R, et al: Exhaled nitric oxide concentrations during treatment of wheezing exacerbations in infants and young children. *Am J Respir Crit Care Med* 1999;159:1284-1288.

104. Patel NR, Hammer J, Nichani S, et al: Effect of inhaled nitric oxide on respiratory mechanics in ventilated infants with RSV bronchiolitis. *Intensive Care Med* 1999;25:81-87.

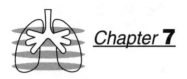

*Chapter **7***

Laboratory Diagnosis

**Daniel E. Noyola, MD,
and Gail J. Demmler, MD**

Departments of Pediatrics and Pathology,
Baylor College of Medicine
and the Diagnostic Virology Laboratory,
Texas Children's Hospital, Houston

The diagnosis of respiratory syncytial virus (RSV) infection can be confirmed by isolating the virus in tissue culture or by detecting the presence of its antigen or nucleic acid in respiratory specimens. RSV is not found in the human body in the absence of recent or current active infection. Therefore, its presence in clinical specimens corroborates a viral etiology for the patient's symptoms. Traditionally, the isolation of RSV in tissue culture has been the method of choice for the clinical confirmation of an infection. However, over the past 2 decades, the development of rapid detection techniques has allowed physicians to obtain an accurate and timely etiologic diagnosis for RSV infections, and to use this information to modify patient management.

Specimen Collection and Handling

To detect the presence of RSV in clinical specimens, it is important to select the appropriate specimen. To effectively isolate RSV, it should be handled in such a way that loss of viral infectivity does not occur during transit to the laboratory. The best specimen for RSV recovery is nasal secretions obtained by either nasal wash or suction.[1-3] This sample reliably produces secretions that contain the infectious virus necessary for culture identification, as well as exfoliated nasopharyngeal cells if viral antigen detection methods are used. Nasal washes can be performed by instilling 1 to 3 mL of sterile saline solution into the patient's nasopharynx through a 5- or 8-French polyethylene catheter, and then applying gentle wall suction to collect the secretions into a DeLee trap, or with a syringe held by hand and attached to the catheter. Alternatively, a tapered bulb-syringe containing 5 to 7 mL of sterile saline solution can be introduced into the patient's nostril until it occludes the nares completely. The bulb should then be squeezed and released quickly,[1] and the nasal wash secretions placed into a separate container for transport to the virology laboratory. The use of nasal swabs is an alternative method for sample collection; cotton-tipped swabs without calcium alginate are recommended.[4] After specimen collection, the swab should be introduced into a vial containing the viral transport media and the shaft cut to close the top of the vial for transport to the laboratory.

The use of a scraper (rhinoprobe) instead of a swab was reported in one study to yield adequate nasopharyngeal cells for viral antigen detection by immunofluorescence testing.[5] Throat swabs and tracheal aspirates yield lower infectious particles and exfoliated cells and, therefore, are not ideal specimens for RSV detection.[6] The virus can also be grown from lung biopsy samples taken from patients with RSV pneumonia.

Specimens should be transported to the laboratory in wet ice as quickly and expeditiously as possible. RSV is a labile virus and does not tolerate changes in temperature, prolonged storage, or transport outside of the body. Heating or freezing the specimen will result in a decreased number of infectious virions in the sample. If specimens cannot be processed rapidly and inoculated into tissue culture within 2 hours of sample collection, they should be kept refrigerated at 4°C. Samples should never be frozen without first consulting the virology laboratory.

The likelihood of identifying RSV as the etiology of a patient's infection is greatest when a specimen is obtained within the first 3 days of the illness, especially when culture isolation is used. Repeat viral cultures or viral antigen detection by immunofluorescence assay (IFA) performed after the initial confirmation of RSV infection will usually become negative by 1 week after onset of illness, in about 50% of patients.[7-9] However, excretion of live virus in some infants has been documented up to 3 weeks after onset of illness.[7] Immunosuppressed patients are also likely to excrete RSV for a longer period.[10,11] In one study, the mean duration of excretion was 16 days for patients receiving chemotherapy and 26 days for patients with immunodeficiencies.[10]

When interpreting laboratory test results for RSV detection, it is also important to take into account the probability that the RSV is associated with the patient's illness. Physicians should be aware of specific regional patterns of RSV activity when considering laboratory confirmation for infection. Although the sensitivity and specificity of a test are characteristics that depend on the test itself, the positive and negative predictive values (ie, the probability that a positive or negative test represents presence or absence of disease for a particular patient) vary according to the prevalence of the disease in a certain population.[12] Particular attention should be paid to the month in which the illness occurs, as well as the patient's geographic region of origin. For example, throughout the United States, RSV epidemics show a marked seasonality, with most positive cultures identified between November and May, and a peak of activity that occurs between December and February.[13-17] In Houston, although RSV can be isolated from clinical specimens year-round, most RSV-containing specimens are obtained between

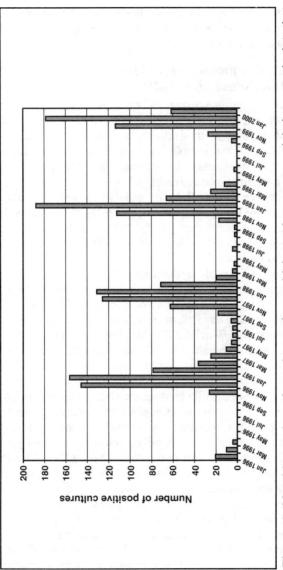

Figure 1: *Monthly number of specimens from which respiratory syncytial virus was isolated at the Diagnostic Virology Laboratory, Texas Children's Hospital in Houston, 1996 to 2000.*

October and April (Figure 1). In contrast, in Hong Kong, the peak incidence of RSV infections occurs in July and August, during the rainy season.[18]

Rapid Diagnostic Techniques for the Detection of RSV

The development of rapid diagnostic techniques for viral detection has received much attention over the last 2 decades. These methods detect viral antigens on the surface of exfoliated nasopharyngeal cells and do not require live virus. Available tests for clinical use include IFA and enzyme immunoassay (EIA).

Direct or indirect IFAs are widely used for rapid diagnosis of RSV infection. The use of monoclonal antibodies in these assays has greatly improved the sensitivity and specificity of the test, both of which are more than 85% in most studies.[19] However, a good specimen containing an adequate number of exfoliated cells is a key factor for a reliable diagnosis with this technique. A greater diagnostic yield by IFA has been consistently found in specimens that have higher numbers of epithelial cells.[2,6] As many as 11% to 31.5% of respiratory specimens submitted to the laboratory for IFA have an inadequate number of cells.[6,20] An appropriate specimen should have at least 100 cells per slide,[21] and the quality of the specimen can be assessed while reading the slide under the microscope. The lack of an immunofluorescence microscope and an inexperienced technician may be limiting factors for some laboratories. However, the high specificity of the IFA and availability of results in 45 minutes to 3 hours (for direct and indirect IFA, respectively) has made the IFA a useful diagnostic technique.

Several commercial membrane EIAs have been developed for the diagnosis of RSV infection (Figure 2). These assays offer the advantages of ease of performance, easy reading of results, and very rapid results (15 to 30 minutes). In fact, these tests can be performed by personnel

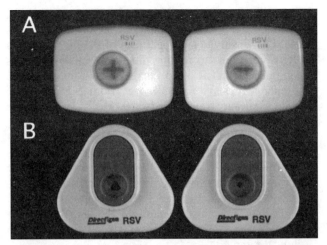

Figure 2: Positive and negative RSV by membrane enzyme immunoassay. A, Abbot TestPack® (Abbott Laboratories, Abbott Park, IL). B, Directigen RSV EIA® (Becton Dickinson, Cockeysville, MD).

with little formal training in virology techniques.[22,23] Another advantage is that they do not require the presence of viable virus to detect an infection, and specimens obtained later in the course of the illness or those with suboptimal handling may yield a positive result, even if viral isolation by culture is negative. Available EIA kits include the Directigen RSV EIA® (Becton Dickinson) and the Abbott TestPack® (Abbott Laboratories). The sensitivity and specificity relative to culture isolation for Directigen EIA® range from 61% to 86.1% and from 69% to 95%, respectively.[24-28] The sensitivity and specificity for the Abbott TestPack® range from 57% to 97% and from 73% to 100%, respectively.[23,24,26-30] It should be noted that nasal washes obtained from preterm infants or from adults and the elderly may not contain sufficient virus to produce a positive rapid antigen test.

Recently, polymerase chain reaction (PCR) has also been used for detection and subtyping of RSV in clinical specimens. The sensitivity and specificity of PCR for detection of RSV compared to routine diagnostic methods varies among different PCR protocols reported in the literature. The reported sensitivity of PCR ranges from 93.5% to 100%, and the specificity from 63.9% to 100%.[31-34] An advantage of this method is its ability to distinguish between RSV types A and B.[34,35] However, the expense of this procedure, and current turn-around time of 8 to 24 hours[36] does not allow for practical use in the clinical laboratory, since faster and less expensive alternatives are available. Nevertheless, it remains a useful tool in the research laboratory, and may have clinical applications in the future if used for the simultaneous detection of several respiratory viruses in 1 clinical sample.[34,37]

Isolation of RSV in Tissue Culture

Isolation of RSV in tissue culture continues to be a useful method for the diagnosis of RSV. To increase the sensitivity for RSV isolation, several cell lines must be inoculated, including a human epithelial (HEP-2, HeLa, or A549 cells), primary monkey kidney, and human fibroblast cell lines.[21,38] It is possible to detect the typical cytopathic effect of RSV (syncytia formation) as early as 2 days of incubation, and most cultures become positive between 2 and 6 days of incubation. A preliminary tentative diagnosis can be made and reported to the clinician on the basis of the characteristic cytopathic effect (Figure 3). Confirmation of a cytopathic effect attributable to RSV is usually performed on infected cells from tissue culture vials using IFA with specific monoclonal antibodies.

The use of shell-vial culture assays decreases the time needed for detection of the virus to 16 hours.[39] The method combines centrifugation to enhance viral attachment to a thin monolayer of cells in culture, and immunofluorescence to detect expression of viral antigens on infected

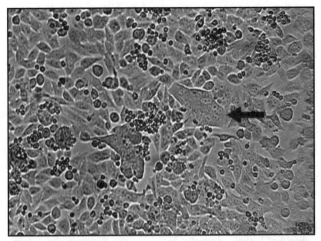

Figure 3: *Characteristic cytopathic effect of respiratory syncytial virus on HEP-2 cell culture. Note the formation of syncytia and wet-sand appearance of infected cells (arrow).*

cells before development of cytopathic effect. The sensitivity and specificity of shell-vial culture compared with conventional culture range from 67.4% to 92.1% and from 82.9% to 100%, respectively.[40-43] Although some laboratories perform shell-vial assays for RSV detection, the labor and expense of this procedure make it less attractive than other rapid diagnostic modalities.

RSV Serology

The diagnosis of RSV infections using serology has no practical application for clinical use. However, the use of serology is useful for epidemiologic studies. Several techniques, including neutralization assays, complement fixation, immunofluorescent antibody testing, and EIA antibody and immunoblot assays, have been developed.[21] It is usually necessary to test acute and convalescent sera and observe an increase in titers to confirm the diagnosis.

Furthermore, assays that detect IgM antibody to RSV show low sensitivity, particularly for infants less than 6 months of age, precluding a definitive diagnosis in a clinically relevant time frame.

Clinical Applications of Viral Diagnosis

The availability of rapid diagnostic assays with a turn-around time as short as 15 minutes makes it possible for clinicians to receive results in a timely fashion and make decisions about patient care. The potential benefits of rapid diagnosis include use of specific antiviral medications, decrease in the use of unnecessary antibiotics, limitation of the use of additional diagnostic tests, and institution of infection control measures.[44,45] The use of rapid viral diagnosis in patients with respiratory tract infections has been shown to decrease the duration of antibiotic use.[45-47] Woo et al reported a reduction in the duration of hospitalization and use of additional laboratory investigations in patients with respiratory infections, after rapid viral diagnosis became available at their hospital.[45] Another effect of the institution of rapid viral diagnosis has been a decrease in hospital costs. Surveys among pediatricians utilizing rapid viral diagnostic tests reported a perception of benefits derived from test results.[45-47] Patients at high risk for complications, such as those with chronic lung or congenital heart disease, may benefit from specific antiviral medications that are prescribed based on rapid identification of RSV infection. Rapid detection of RSV can also be used as part of an infection control program to decrease nosocomial RSV transmission.[48-50] For example, during an RSV outbreak in a neonatal intensive care unit, IFA was used to rapidly identify and isolate infected infants to control the outbreak.[51]

It has recently been reported that infants with congenital heart disease who are subjected to heart surgery close to the onset of an RSV infection may have a greater mortality.[52] Rapid diagnostic assays can be used to screen infants before elective surgery, and those with a positive RSV rapid test can have their surgery postponed to avoid possible complications in the postoperative period.[53] Other possible benefits to using rapid tests for RSV diagnosis are more difficult to measure, and include patients' and families' emotional relief, and increased confidence in the physician.

References

1.   Hall CB, Douglas RG Jr: Clinically useful method for the isolation of respiratory syncytial virus. *J Infect Dis* 1975;131:1-5.

2.   Ahluwalia G, Embree J, McNicol P, et al: Comparison of nasopharyngeal aspirate and nasopharyngeal swab specimens for respiratory syncytial virus diagnosis by cell culture, indirect immunofluorescence assay, and enzyme-linked immunosorbent assay. *J Clin Microbiol* 1987;25:763-767.

3.   Masters HB, Weber KO, Groothuis JR, et al: Comparison of nasopharyngeal washings and swab specimens for diagnosis of respiratory syncytial virus by EIA, FAT, and cell culture. *Diagn Microbiol Infect Dis* 1987;8:101-105.

4.   Frayha H, Castriciano S, Mahony J, et al: Nasopharyngeal swabs and nasopharyngeal aspirates equally effective for the diagnosis of viral respiratory disease in hospitalized children. *J Clin Microbiol* 1989;27:1387-1389.

5.   Jalowayski AA, Walpita P, Puryear BA, et al: Rapid detection of respiratory syncytial virus in nasopharyngeal specimens obtained with the rhinoprobe scraper. *J Clin Microbiol* 1990;28:738-741.

6.   Treuhaft MW, Soukup JM, Sullivan BJ: Practical recommendations for the detection of pediatric respiratory syncytial virus infections. *J Clin Microbiol* 1985;22:270-273.

7.   Hall CB, Douglas RG Jr, Geiman JM: Respiratory syncytial virus infections in infants: quantitation and duration of shedding. *J Pediatr* 1976;89:11-15.

8.   McIntosh K, Hendry RM, Fahnestock ML, et al: Enzyme-linked immunosorbent assay for detection of respiratory syncytial virus infection: application to clinical samples. *J Clin Microbiol* 1982;16:329-333.

9. Mackie PL, Madge PJ, Getty S, et al: Rapid diagnosis of respiratory syncytial virus infection by using nasal swabs. *J Clin Microbiol* 1991;29:2653-2655.

10. Hall CB, Powell KR, MacDonald NE, et al: Respiratory syncytial viral infection in children with compromised immune function. *N Engl J Med* 1986;315:77-81.

11. King JC Jr, Burke AR, Clemens JD, et al: Respiratory syncytial virus illnesses in human immunodeficiency virus- and noninfected children. *Pediatr Infect Dis J* 1993;12:733-739.

12. Shapiro ED: Epidemiology and biostatistics. In: Feigin RD, Cherry JD, eds. *Textbook of Pediatric Infectious Diseases*, 4th ed. Philadelphia, WB Saunders, 1998, pp 2907-2921.

13. Glezen WP, Paredes A, Taber LH: Influenza in children. Relationship to other respiratory agents. *JAMA* 1980;243:1345-1349.

14. Denny FW, Clyde WA Jr: Acute lower respiratory tract infections in nonhospitalized children. *J Pediatr* 1986;108:635-646.

15. Dagan R, Hall CB, Powell KR, et al: Epidemiology and laboratory diagnosis of infection with viral and bacterial pathogens in infants hospitalized for suspected sepsis. *J Pediatr* 1989;115:351-356.

16. Hendry RM, Pierik LT, McIntosh K: Prevalence of respiratory syncytial virus subgroups over six consecutive outbreaks: 1981-1987. *J Infect Dis* 1989;160:185-190.

17. Gilchrist S, Török TJ, Gary HE Jr, et al: National surveillance for respiratory syncytial virus, United States, 1985-1990. *J Infect Dis* 1994;170:986-990.

18. Sung RY, Murray HG, Chan RC, et al: Seasonal patterns of respiratory syncytial virus infection in Hong Kong: a preliminary report. *J Infect Dis* 1987;156:527-528.

19. Kellogg JA: Culture vs direct antigen assays for detection of microbial pathogens from lower respiratory tract specimens suspected of containing the respiratory syncytial virus. *Arch Pathol Lab Med* 1991;115:451-458.

20. Fulton RE, Middleton PJ: Comparison of immunofluorescence and isolation techniques in the diagnosis of respiratory viral infections of children. *Infect Immun* 1974;10:92-101.

21. Tristram DA, Welliver RC: Respiratory syncytial virus. In: Lennette EH, Lennette DA, Lennette ET, eds. *Diagnostic Procedures for Viral, Rickettsial and Chlamydial Infections*, 7th ed. Washington, DC, American Public Health Association, 1995, pp 539-552.

22. Subbarao EK, Dietrich MC, De Sierra TM, et al: Rapid detection of respiratory syncytial virus by a biotin-enhanced immunoassay: test performance by laboratory technologists and housestaff. *Pediatr Infect Dis J* 1989;8:865-869.

23. Krilov LR, Lipson SM, Barone SR, et al: Evaluation of a rapid diagnostic test for respiratory syncytial virus (RSV): potential for bedside diagnosis. *Pediatrics* 1994;93:903-906.

24. Michaels MG, Serdy C, Barbadora K, et al: Respiratory syncytial virus: a comparison of diagnostic modalities. *Pediatr Infect Dis J* 1992;11:613-616.

25. Waner JL, Whitehurst NJ, Todd SJ, et al: Comparison of Directigen RSV® with viral isolation and direct immunofluorescence for the identification of respiratory syncytial virus. *J Clin Microbiol* 1990;28:480-483.

26. Halstead DC, Todd S, Fritch G: Evaluation of five methods for respiratory syncytial virus detection. *J Clin Microbiol* 1990;28:1021-1025.

27. Rothbarth PH, Hermus MC, Schrijnemakers P: Reliability of two new test kits for rapid diagnosis of respiratory syncytial virus infection. *J Clin Microbiol* 1991;29:824-826.

28. Dominguez EA, Taber LH, Couch RB: Comparison of rapid diagnostic techniques for respiratory syncytial and influenza A virus respiratory infections in young children. *J Clin Microbiol* 1993;31:2286-2290.

29. Wren CG, Bate BJ, Masters HB, et al: Detection of respiratory syncytial virus antigen in nasal washings by Abbott TestPack® enzyme immunoassay. *J Clin Microbiol* 1990;28:1395-1397.

30. Thomas EE, Book LE: Comparison of two rapid methods for detection of respiratory syncytial virus (RSV) (TestPack RSV® and Ortho RSV ELISA®) with direct immunofluorescence and virus isolation for the diagnosis of pediatric RSV infection. *J Clin Microbiol* 1991;29:632-635.

31. Freymuth F, Eugene G, Vabret A, et al: Detection of respiratory syncytial virus by reverse transcription-PCR and hybridization with a DNA enzyme immunoassay. *J Clin Microbiol* 1995;33:3352-3355.

32. Henkel JH, Aberle SW, Kundi M, et al: Improved detection of respiratory syncytial virus in nasal aspirates by seminested RT-PCR. *J Med Virol* 1997;53:366-371.

33. Eugene-Ruellan G, Freymuth F, Bahloul C, et al: Detection of respiratory syncytial virus A and B and parainfluenzavirus 3 sequences in respiratory tracts of infants by a single PCR with primers targeted to the L-polymerase gene and differential hybridization. *J Clin Microbiol* 1998;36:796-801.

34. Stockton J, Ellis JS, Saville M, et al: Multiplex PCR for typing and subtyping influenza and respiratory syncytial viruses. *J Clin Microbiol* 1998;36:2990-2995.

35. Gottschalk J, Zbinden R, Kaempf L, et al: Discrimination of respiratory syncytial virus subgroups A and B by reverse transcription-PCR. *J Clin Microbiol* 1996;34:41-43.

36. Paton AW, Paton JC, Lawrence AJ, et al: Rapid detection of respiratory syncytial virus in nasopharyngeal aspirates by reverse transcription and polymerase chain reaction amplification. *J Clin Microbiol* 1992;30:901-904.

37. Gröndahl B, Puppe W, Hoppe A, et al: Rapid identification of nine microorganisms causing acute respiratory tract infections by single-tube multiplex reverse transcription-PCR: feasibility study. *J Clin Microbiol* 1999;37:1-7.

38. Arens MQ, Swierkosz EM, Schmidt RR, et al: Enhanced isolation of respiratory syncytial virus in cell culture. *J Clin Microbiol* 1986;23:800-802.

39. Smith MC, Creutz C, Huang YT: Detection of respiratory syncytial virus in nasopharyngeal secretions by shell vial technique. *J Clin Microbiol* 1991;29:463-465.

40. Johnston SL, Siegel CS: Evaluation of direct immunofluorescence, enzyme immunoassay, centrifugation culture, and conventional culture for the detection of respiratory syncytial virus. *J Clin Microbiol* 1990;28:2394-2397.

41. Meziere A, Mollat C, Lapied R, et al: Detection of respiratory syncytial virus antigen after 72 hours of culture. *J Med Virol* 1990;31:241-244.

42. Lee SH, Boutilier JE, MacDonald MA, et al: Enhanced detection of respiratory viruses using the shell vial technique and monoclonal antibodies. *J Virol Methods* 1992;39:39-46.

43. Shih SR, Tsao KC, Ning HC, et al: Diagnosis of respiratory tract viruses in 24 h by immunofluorescent staining of shell vial cultures containing Madin-Darby Canine Kidney (MDCK) cells. *J Virol Methods* 1999;81:77-81.

44. Richman DD, Cleveland PH, Redfield DC, et al: Rapid viral diagnosis. *J Infect Dis* 1984;149:298-310.

45. Woo PC, Chiu SS, Seto WH, et al: Cost-effectiveness of rapid diagnosis of viral respiratory tract infections in pediatric patients. *J Clin Microbiol* 1997;35:1579-1581.

46. Carlsen KH, Ørstavik I: Respiratory syncytial virus infections in Oslo 1972-1978. II. Clinical and laboratory studies. *Acta Paediatr Scand* 1980;69:723-729.

47. Adcock PM, Stout GG, Hauck MA, et al: Effect of rapid viral diagnosis on the management of children hospitalized with lower respiratory tract infection. *Pediatr Infect Dis J* 1997;16:842-846.

48. Beekmann SE, Engler HD, Collins AS, et al: Rapid identification of respiratory viruses: impact on isolation practices and transmission among immunocompromised pediatric patients. *Infect Control Hosp Epidemiol* 1996;17:581-586.

49. Doherty JA, Brookfield DS, Gray J, et al: Cohorting of infants with respiratory syncytial virus. *J Hosp Infect* 1998;38:203-206.

50. Karanfil LV, Conlon M, Lykens K, et al: Reducing the rate of nosocomially transmitted respiratory syncytial virus. *Am J Infect Control* 1999;27:91-96.

51. Mintz L, Ballard RA, Sniderman SH, et al: Nosocomial respiratory syncytial virus infections in an intensive care nursery: rapid diagnosis by direct immunofluorescence. *Pediatrics* 1979;64:149-153.

52. Khongphatthanayothin A, Wong PC, Samara Y, et al: Impact of respiratory syncytial virus infection on surgery for congenital heart disease: postoperative course and outcome. *Crit Care Med* 1999;27:1974-1981.

53. Altman CA, Englund JA, Demmler GJ, et al: Respiratory syncytial virus in patients with congenital heart disease: a contemporary look at epidemiology and success of preoperative screening. *Pediatr Cardiol* 2000;21:433-438.

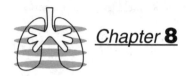

Chapter 8

Therapy of RSV

William J. Rodriguez, MD

Professor of Pediatrics,
Division of Pediatric Infectious Diseases
George Washington University School of Medicine,
Children's National Medical Center, Washington, DC

I n treating patients with respiratory syncytial virus (RSV) infection, it is important to know that other clinical conditions can mimic it, even though the epidemiologic data, time of year, and affected age group may suggest that the bronchiolitic manifestations are secondary to RSV. Importantly, the clinical condition of those patients at risk may progress from what appears to be an asymptomatic state to a full respiratory deterioration with no previous signs of upper respiratory tract infection. Most patients with RSV infection do not need to be hospitalized. Once the diagnosis is made, the main outpatient treatment is supportive. The elements of home supportive care include oral hydration, feeding, and maintaining close contact between the parent and the caregiver. In some special situations, the use of supplemental oxygen at home is acceptable.[1,2]

Hypoxemia is probably one of the most serious results of bronchiolitis. The primary physiologic abnormality in RSV bronchiolitis with hypoxemia is a disturbance of the ventilation to perfusion ratio, and relatively low concentrations of supplemental oxygen are usually sufficient to correct the problem. It is critical that the physician monitor the use of oxygen, or at least confirm the need for oxygen by pulse oximetry.

In some studies, the correlation of physical findings, such as cyanosis and rales or crackles, with arterial oxygen has been good. However, other physical findings, such as heart rate and respiratory rate, have not correlated as well. In most situations where lower respiratory tract involvement is suspected, pulse oximetry is reliable. However, this method may not be available in all instances. Also, mistakes can occur, such as when the sensor is not applied directly to the skin or when it detaches from the skin. Other factors that may adversely affect the findings of pulse oximetry include hypothermia with some peripheral vasoconstriction, low blood pressure, and anemia. It is also important for the clinician to remember that, for oxygen saturation below 80%, the monitors may not be accurate.[3]

Supportive Outpatient Management

The treatment of RSV bronchiolitis is primarily symptomatic. For those managed in the outpatient setting, it is important to maintain adequate hydration. Since RSV bronchiolitis usually does not dehydrate a child, clinicians must remember that aggressive hydration in the face of increased production of antidiuretic hormone (ADH) could result in hyponatremia and seizures. Seizures in patients with RSV, particularly in those with hypercarbia or those needing ventilatory assistance, have been reported in the literature.[4,5] Thus, it is important for the clinician to monitor or to advise the parent about fluid intake. Additionally, as some have reported, aspiration can occur in RSV patients while they are being fed,[6] contributing to or worsening the respiratory status of the patient. The use of aminophylline is contraindicated.[7]

Supportive Inpatient Management

Approximately 1% of previously healthy children with RSV are hospitalized. The decision for hospitalization should be made based on at least 1 of 3 factors: historical, clinical, or laboratory/radiology test results. Historically, the age of a child (< 3 months), the degree of prematurity (< 34 weeks), or the presence of chronic lung disease were used as reasons for hospitalization. A clinically based decision depends on the presence of clinical common sense findings, such as toxic appearance, a respiratory rate of 70 beats per minute, or the degree of wheezing/respiratory distress. The third set of factors appears more objective, and depends on specific laboratory/radiographic findings, such as oxygen saturation ≤95% or the presence of atelectasis on radiographic examination. In addition, observations such as pulsus paradoxus, pallor, and lethargy are also important to consider. Additionally, an increasing carbon dioxide tension ($PACO_2$) ≥ 40 mm Hg is considered a disturbing finding, suggestive of impending respiratory insufficiency. Other factors include the distance between the patient's home and the hospital, and the capability of the parent to follow instructions and deliver the care.[8-11]

For patients who require hospitalization, an important supportive measure is providing warm, humidified, supplemental O_2 by headbox or tent, one of the most reliable ways to treat the hypoxemia of bronchiolitis. Clinicians should strive to maintain saturation at a minimum of 92%.[3,12] Calculation of parenteral fluids depends on the assessment of the particular patient. If the child is able to take fluids, parenteral fluids may be run at two thirds maintenance[13]; it is key to try to prevent not only pulmonary congestion in patients such as those with congenital heart disease, but also to pay appropriate attention to the possibility that with inappropriate ADH secretion, overhydration may worsen the situation. Feeding those patients with high respiratory rates (60 to 70 beats per minute) can be associated with difficulties, ultimately resulting in vomiting and, even, aspiration. Very sick children with high respiratory rates or apnea should receive intravenous fluids only. In considering caloric replacement, the concerns of oral feeding were addressed earlier, particularly in view of the risk of aspiration. Since the signs of aspiration and bronchiolitis may be indistinguishable from one another, the clinician must initiate feeds cautiously to try to avoid such complications.[6]

In hospitalized patients, clinicians must closely follow heart rate, respiratory rate, input and output, electrolytes, and pulse oximetry. The presence of severe oxygen desaturation, acidosis, or recurrent apneic episodes should lead to consideration of ventilatory assistance or monitoring in an intensive care unit (ICU).[12,13] Providing oxygen at a concentration of 40% usually helps to maintain the $PACO_2$ between 70 and 90 mm Hg. The caregiver must be aware of the contribution of the factors mentioned earlier, such as acidosis, anemia, and shunting, and some patients may require additional supplemental oxygen. Following the carbon dioxide level is also important.

Respiratory failure should be considered if the infant develops a $PACO_2$ that exceeds 55 mm Hg, if the PAO_2 falls below 70 mm Hg while 60% supplemental oxygen is being administered, or if the infant develops acidosis.[14] In such instances, the patient should be transferred to the pediatric ICU and mechanical ventilation should be considered.[11] Patients who continue to deteriorate despite maximum ventilatory support have been successfully supported with extracorporeal membrane oxygenation (ECMO). Although the duration of ECMO support has been somewhat longer for patients with RSV than for conventional neonatal ventilatory indications, the neurologic outcome has been excellent in the survivors.[13]

Symptomatic Therapy: Bronchodilators

The use of bronchodilators with various mechanisms of action is widely accepted in the United States, although not necessarily in other countries. Bronchodilators with various mechanisms of action have been used in patients with RSV bronchiolitis, including α-adrenergic agents, such as phenylephrine and phenylpropanolamine, β_2-adrenergic agents, such as albuterol, and anticholinergic bronchodilators. When examining the performance of such agents, one finds ongoing controversies about the benefit of each. Studies by Alario et al, Klassen et al, and Schuh et al[15-17] report beneficial effect, although indeterminate effect was shown in other studies.[18,19] In one study, some negative effects of bronchodilators were observed.[20] Investigators such as McBride[21] suggest that there may be a subset of patients who respond to β_2-adrenergic agonists. Such patients can be identified by their response to treatment with β_2-agonists in the emergency department, and may not even need to be admitted to the hospital. Additionally, McBride states that the dose used in most clinical studies of 0.15 mg/kg is lower than what he used (essentially, a 2.5-mg unit dose for infants), raising the possibility that some infants are being undertreated. Concerns about the use of β_2-adrenergics include side effects such as exacerbation of respiratory symptoms, (ie, hypoxemia or airway obstruction). These agents may alter the ventilation and perfusion in patients with severe RSV, who then experience the paradoxical effect of increased airway obstruction.[22] This latter effect may very well be the result of decreased bronchial muscle tone in patients with floppy airways, such as children with tracheal malacia or bronchomalacia. Thus, β_2-adrenergic bronchodilators may be partially effective in some patients, but the patients need to be observed very closely for side effects.

α-Adrenergic agents may be more effective than β_2-adrenergics in terms of their clinical scores.[21] Among this latter group, α-adrenergics, such as phenylephrine and phenylpropanolamine, as well as agents such as epinephrine, which has both α- and β_2-adrenergic agonist activity, showed favorable results. In one study, Menon et al compared epinephrine to albuterol.[23] Patients received a dose at 0 and 30 minutes of either 3 mL of a 5 mg/mL solution of albuterol (Ventolin®, 1.5 mg combined with 2.7 mL of 0.9% saline solution to make a total of 3 mL), or 3 mL of 1:1000 epinephrine (adrenaline solution, 3 mg by nebulizer) with continuous flow oxygen at 5 to 6 minutes. The outcome was the probability of emergency department discharge. The mean percent oxygen saturation at 60 minutes was significantly higher in the epinephrine group, with only 33% of the patients admitted to the hospital, compared with 81% of the albuterol group, a significant difference.

Epinephrine, which has both α- and β_2-adrenergic activity, was more efficient in eliciting a favorable clinical response in children under 1 year of age, who had no previous history of wheezing and who were observed in the emergency department. Those who received epinephrine were more likely to be discharged earlier. The patients on albuterol had higher heart rates, while patients with epinephrine had increased pallor. Another study examined the use of epinephrine administered subcutaneously compared to placebo (saline), and found that epinephrine produced dramatic improvement in clinical score for almost all infants with bronchiolitis.[24] Although the data are controversial, it is likely that there exists a group of children with bronchiolitis who will respond to nebulized bronchodilator therapy; such treatment may be necessary for 24 to 48 hours. This group includes those with underlying bronchopulmonary dysplasia (now known as chronic lung disease of prematurity) or reactive airway disease. There have been anecdotal reports on the use of aerosolized bronchodilators after hospital discharge for those who responded to inpatient therapy.

The use of anticholinergic bronchodilators for a first episode of bronchiolitis and the use of corticosteroids in serious RSV disease appear to be unsubstantiated in many studies.[25-28]

Antivirals

The only FDA-approved antiviral preparation for RSV is ribavirin (Virazole®).[29] Ribavirin is a broad-spectrum agent with activity against both the orthomyxoviruses and the paramyxoviruses, such as influenza viruses (both A and B), on one hand, and the measles virus and RSV on the other. Ribavirin is a synthetic purine nucleoside analogue of guanosine that is not virucidal, but virustatic, whose mechanism of action is inhibition of the efficiency of translation of viral mRNA into viral structural proteins, resulting in the suppression of viral RNA polymerase activity. This action results in interference with the viral mRNA expression and, ultimately, with protein synthesis. To date, no ribavirin-resistant RSV strains have been observed.[25] Additionally, it has been shown that, in vivo, ribavirin reduces the RSV IgE response. It is important to remember that RSV titers usually peak within 3 days of onset of bronchiolitis symptoms. This usually occurs within 10 days following initial exposure to the virus. Because its mechanism of action is inhibition of viral replication during the active replication phase,[30] the earlier ribavirin is used during the course of acute infection, the more likely it is to have an effect.

Despite the existence of many studies, controversy about benefits vs cost of ribavirin therapy continues.[31-40] Two studies that dealt with the use of ribavirin in mechanically ventilated children illustrate this controversy. Smith et al reported that when mechanically ventilated children with severe RSV disease received either ribavirin or a placebo (water), children on ribavirin had a shorter duration of mechanical ventilation and less need for supplemental oxygen and hospitalization.[31] A more recent study conducted by Meert et al compared ribavirin with a placebo (saline), and failed to find a decrease in days of mechanical ventilation, oxygen supplementation, ICU stay, or hospitalization.[37] There are major methodologic differences between the 2 studies that could account for the observed differences. For example, the use of sterile distilled water in the control group in one of the studies could have led to the adverse effect on the overall reactivity in the placebo group. However, when the amount of water that could have reached the bronchioles is examined, the amount is found to be infinitesimally low compared to that which was used to produce such bronchospastic changes. There were also differences in the mean age of the subjects and in underlying disorders, which may account for some of the discrepancies. Therefore, the question of ribavirin efficacy in mechanically ventilated children remains unanswered.

In 1996, the American Academy of Pediatrics suggested that ribavirin could be considered for treatment of hospitalized infants and children with severe lower respiratory infection (LRI) caused by RSV.[41] The clinician should carefully weigh the benefits of its use in high-risk patients, such as those with congenital heart disease, chronic lung disease, or other chronic diseases. Others who might be considered candidates for ribavirin treatment are previously healthy premature infants, infants who have underlying immunosuppressive diseases or are receiving immunosuppressive therapy, or those who may have neurologic or neuromuscular problems, such as cerebral palsy or myasthenia gravis, which may also put them at risk.

Some difficulties with ribavirin administration stem from the fact that it must be administered with a machine called a SPAG2 unit, which should only be operated by trained personnel. Additionally, ribavirin should only be administered in a well-ventilated, negative-pressure room. There is also a recommendation for caregivers to wear a respiratory, not a surgical, mask. Ribavirin should not be administered with other aerosols, and there is a warning that pregnant women should not be exposed to aerosol.

Part of the controversy for ribavirin treatment may arise from the fact that pharmacologic outcome analyses that are now routinely used in the evaluation of studies, were not part of some of the studies conducted in the 1980s. Cost-benefit analyses for ribavirin therapy are not available. Ribavirin is used at 20 mg/mL of diluent and is administered for 12 to 18 hours daily for 3 to 7 days. The aerosol particles are 1 to 2 μm in diameter and should be small enough to reach the lower respiratory tract.[42] In a recent study, Englund et al used triple the concentration of ribavirin over a shorter period of time, 60 mg/mL of diluent for 2 hours, 3 times daily.[43] The clinical results were comparable in both short- and long-term ribavirin therapies that delivered the same total daily dose. This approach could conceivably reduce the number of hours that patients would be exposed, and, therefore, reduce the time that the support staff would be exposed.

Antimicrobials

As a rule, bronchiolitis is a self-limited viral process. The findings of Hall et al that association of bacterial infections occured in 2% or less of 565 hospitalized children suggest that the use of antimicrobials in such populations is seldom indicated.[44] Nevertheless, if one suspects bacterial superinfection in children—as manifested by high white blood cell counts, dropping platelet counts, recurrent apnea, circulatory impairment, impressive lobar changes on x-ray, or positive cultures—antimicrobial therapy should be considered.[3]

Immunotherapy

When clinicians consider the reasons for the severity of RSV disease, the answer appears to be that RSV antibodies may not completely protect against infection and reinfection. More importantly, the severity of RSV lower respiratory tract infections and disease inversely correlates with the presence of RSV neutralizing antibodies. Investigators reported that titers between 1:300 and 1:400 in infants are protective. Such titers are similar to those observed in the cotton rat model described in Chapter 3.[45-48]

Hence, it was speculated that serum antibody may be useful in the treatment of serious RSV LRI.[45]

In 1985, a study was conducted in which patients who had been hospitalized with RSV LRI were treated with 2 g/kg of IV immunoglobulin that had RSV neutralizing titers of 1:5,000.[49] After administration of these doses, the resulting antibody titers rose from a mean of 114 to 877, compared to 119 in control infants. It was also demonstrated in the subsequent 24-hour period that the oxygen saturation improved significantly in intravenous immunoglobulin (IGIV)-treated patients, when compared to controls. A significant reduction of viral titers in respiratory secretions by day 2 in treated vs control patients was also demonstrated. Increased T and B lymphocyte counts were also observed. In follow-up studies, the presence of RSV IgG neutralizing antibodies 6 weeks after discharge was looked for, and the antibody response against DPT after a second DPT shot, and 6 weeks after the third DPT shot, were assessed. No evidence of immune suppression was observed in T and B cell lymphocyte counts and functional studies. A 1-year follow-up study demonstrated no increased evidence of susceptibility to RSV infection or to other respiratory infections. Although antibody titers were somewhat lower in those who received the RSV-IGIV, all children had titers that were measurable and not significantly different from controls.

Therapeutic studies that used a preparation with high-titer IgG antibodies against RSV (RSV-IGIV, RespiGam™) both in previously healthy and high-risk patients, compared to controls, were subsequently conducted.[50-51] Both those children who were previously healthy and those children at risk for serious RSV infection were matched against controls, and received 1,500 mg/kg of RSV-IGIV or plasma placebo. Treated children demonstrated RSV-neutralizing titers as high as 1:1,422 after infusion. Viral eradication of RSV from the nasopharyngeal sites occurred in 48 to 72 hours after administration of the RSV-IGIV, both in a high-risk population (gestational age < 32 weeks, with chronic lung disease or congenital heart disease) and in the previously healthy population. However, there was no significant difference in reduction in days for RSV hospitalization, stay in the ICU, or duration of mechanical ventilation. Study patients were followed for 1 year after their hospitalization, and failed to develop any increase in RSV LRI severity upon subsequent reinfection. In summary, although RSV-IGIV was safe and as effective as the earlier standard polyclonal preparation in reducing RSV in the nasopharynx, no treatment efficacy was observed.[50,51]

A monoclonal antibody preparation that was shown to have excellent anti-RSV activity in mice,[52] palivizumab (Synagis™), has been recently developed. Palivizumab demonstrates broad neutralization activity against RSV isolates in the mouse model, and was found to be 50 to 100 times more potent compared to RSV-IGIV.[53] The safety of palivizumab was demonstrated in adult volunteers. In a small study of treated children ventilated less than 24 hours, a reduction in virus load in the tracheal aspirates was observed, and was significantly different from similarly infected controls.[54] However, no difference in the number of days of hospitalization, in mechanical ventilation days, or in the need for supplemental oxygen was noted. This study did not have access to the latter clinical information. In a larger study conducted in the United States and Panama, no significant differences in outcome between the palivizumab-treated and untreated groups were observed, although palivizumab was observed to be safe.[55] Adverse effects seen with palivizumab were not significant. The presence of erythema, pain, and induration or adverse event rates did not differ from the placebo group. However, in both studies, the number of patients may have been too small to detect any significant differences. Based on the data that are now available, palivizumab should not be used for the treatment of RSV.

Animal studies suggest that reduction of viral shedding may not be sufficient to alter the magnitude of inflammatory response after RSV infection, and that the use of antiviral agents, such as palivizumab, should be combined with an immune modulator.[56-59] Performance results in human populations are pending.

Infection Control

The best way of handling RSV disease is to prevent it, and it is important for caregivers to realize that prevention is an important way of preventing morbidity. The infection rate within a hospital may exceed 26%; thus, the education of caregivers, particularly in the area of hand-washing, is critical. It was demonstrated that the use of rapid virus identification tests and cohort of nursing support can reduce the nosocomial infection rate to 9%. In our institution, the nosocomial rate was decreased from 25% to 2% when patients were screened for RSV infection on admission, and when RSV-positive children were cohorted to a specific ward with dedicated nursing staff.

Immunotherapy in Transplant Recipients

Transplant recipients were found to benefit from immunotherapy when it was used as part of combination therapy.[59-62] Patients recovering from bone marrow or solid organ transplants may be at high risk for RSV LRT infection and pneumonitis, and may experience diffuse alveolar damage and death. In the experience of Whimbey et al,[61,62] as well as others, combining ribavirin and RSV-IGIV results in significant clinical improvement and improved survival. Hence, immunotherapy combined with antiviral activity appears to result in a beneficial response. Randomized controlled trials are needed to develop further recommendations in this area.

References

1. Darville T, Yamauchi T: Respiratory syncytial virus. *Pediatr Rev* 1998;19:55-61.

2. Welliver RC, Ogra PL: *Infectious Diseases*, 2nd ed. Philadelphia, WB Saunders Co, 1998, pp 2148-2156.

3. Rakshi K, Couriel JM: Management of acute bronchiolitis. *Arch Dis Child* 1994;71:463-469.

4. Rivers RP, Forsling ML, Oliver RP: Inappropriate secretions of antidiuretic hormone in infants with respiratory infections. *Arch Dis Child* 1981;56:358-363.

5. van Steensell-Moll HA, Hazelzet JA, van der Voort E, et al: Excessive secretion of antidiuretic hormone in infections with respiratory syncytial virus. *Arch Dis Child* 1990,65:1237-1239.

6. Khoshoo V, Edell D: Previously healthy infants may have increased risk of aspiration during respiratory syncytial viral bronchiolitis. *Pediatrics* 1999;104:1389-1390.

7. Brooks LJ, Cropp GJ: Theophylline therapy in bronchiolitis. A retrospective study. *Am J Dis Child* 1981;135:934-936.

8. Horst PS: Bronchiolitis. *Am Fam Physician* 1994;49:1449-1453,1456.

9. Shaw KN, Bell LM, Sherman NH: Outpatient assessment of patients with bronchiolitis. *Am J Dis Child* 1991;145:151-155.

10. Mulholland EK, Olinsky A, Shann FA: Clinical findings and severity of acute bronchiolitis. *Lancet* 1990;335:1259-1261.

11. Moylett EH, Piedra PA: Respiratory syncytial virus infection: diagnosis, treatment and prevention. *Hosp Med* 1999;35:10-17.

12. Hall CB, McCarthy CA: Respiratory syncytial virus. In: Mandell GL, Bennett JE, Dolin R, eds. *Principles and Practices of Infectious Diseases*, 4th ed. New York, Churchill Livingstone, 1995, pp 1501-1508.

13. Steinhorn RH, Green TP: Use of extracorporeal membrane oxygenation in the treatment of respiratory syncytial virus bronchiolitis: the national experience, 1983 to1988. *J Pediatr* 1990; 116:338-342.

14. Rodriguez WJ, Parrott RH: Ribavirin aerosol treatment of serious respiratory syncytial virus infection in infants. *Infect Dis Clin North Am* 1987;1:425-439.

15. Alario AJ, Lewander WJ, Dennehy P, et al: The efficacy of nebulized metaproterenol in wheezing infants and young children. *Am J Dis Child* 1992;146:412-418.

16. Klassen TP, Rowe PC, Sutcliffe T, et al: Randomized trial of salbutamol in acute bronchiolitis. *J Pediatr* 1991;118:807-811.

17. Schuh S, Canny G, Reisman JJ, et al: Nebulized albuterol in acute bronchiolitis. *J Pediatr* 1990;117:633-637.

18. Gadomski AM, Lichenstein R, Horton L, et al: Efficacy of albuterol in the management of bronchiolitis. *Pediatrics* 1994;93:907-912.

19. Wang EE, Milner R, Allen U, et al: Bronchodilators for treatment of mild bronchiolitis; a factorial randomised trial. *Arch Dis Child* 1992;67:289-293.

20. Ho L, Collis G, Landau LI, et al: Effect of salbutamol on oxygen saturation in bronchiolitis *Arch Dis Child* 1991;66:1061-1064.

21. McBride J: Is there a role for bronchodilators and corticosteroids in the management of acute RSV lower respiratory tract infections? In: Hiatt PW, ed. *RSV and Asthma: Is There a Link?* New York, American Thoracic Society, 1998, pp 34-39.

22. Prendiville A, Green S, Silverman M: Paradoxical response to nebulised salbutamol in wheezy infants, assessed by partial expiratory flow-volume curves. *Thorax* 1987;42:86-91.

23. Menon K, Sutcliffe T, Klassen TP: A randomized trial comparing the efficacy of epinephrine with salbutamol in the treatment of acute bronchiolitis. *J Pediatr* 1995;126:1004-1007.

24. Lowell DI, Lister G, Von Koss H, et al: Wheezing in infants: the response to epinephrine *Pediatrics* 1987;79:939-945.

25. Lugo RA, Nahata MC: Pathogenesis and treatment of bronchiolitis. *Clin Pharm* 1993;12:95-116.

26. Springer C, Bar-Yishay E, Uwayyed K, et al: Corticosteroids do not affect the clinical or physiological status of infants with bronchiolitis. *Pediatr Pulmonol* 1990;9:181-185.

27. Wang EE, Milner R, Allen U, et al: Bronchodilators for treatment of mild bronchiolitis: a factorial randomised trial. *Arch Dis Child* 1992;67:289-293.

28. Roosevelt G, Sheehan K, Grupp-Phelan J, et al: Dexamethasone in bronchiolitis: a randomised controlled trial. *Lancet* 1996;348:292-295.

29. *Physicians' Desk Reference*, 53rd ed. Montvale, NJ, Medical Economics Co, 1999, pp 1382-1384.

30. McIntosh K, Chanock RM: Respiratory syncytial virus. In: Fields BN, Knipe DM, Chanock RM, et al, eds. *Virology*, 2nd ed. New York, Raven Press, 1990, pp 1045-1072.

31. Smith DW, Frankel LR, Mathers LH, et al: A controlled trial of aerosolized ribavirin in infants receiving mechanical ventilation for severe respiratory syncytial virus infection. *N Engl J Med* 1991;325:24-29.

32. Hall CB, McBride JT, Walsh EE, et al: Aerosolized ribavirin treatment of infants with respiratory syncytial virus infection. A randomized double-blind study. *N Engl J Med* 1983;308:1443-1447.

33. Hall CB, McBride JT, Gala CL, et al: Ribavirin treatment of respiratory syncytial viral infection in infants with underlying cardiopulmonary disease. *JAMA* 1985;254:3047-3051.

34. Rodriguez WJ, Kim HW, Brandt CD, et al: Aerosolized ribavirin in the treatment of patients with respiratory syncytial virus disease. *Pediatr Infect Dis J* 1987;6:159-163.

35. Groothuis JR, Woodin KA, Katz R, et al: Early ribavirin treatment of respiratory syncytial viral infection in high-risk children. *J Pediatr* 1990;117:792-798.

36. Hiatt PW, Treece D, Morris L, et al: Longitudinal pulmonary function (PF) following treatment with ribavirin in infants hospitalized with RSV bronchiolitis [abstract]. *Am J Respir Crit Care Med* 1994;179:A354.

37. Meert KL, Sarnaik AP, Gelmini MJ, et al: Aerosolized ribavirin in mechanically ventilated children with respiratory syncytial virus lower respiratory tract disease: a prospective, double-blind, randomized trial. *Crit Care Med* 1994;22:566-572.

38. Wheeler JG, Wofford J, Turner RB: Historical cohort evaluation of ribavirin efficacy in respiratory syncytial virus infection. *Pediatr Infect Dis J* 1993;12:209-213.

39. Janai HK, Stutman HR, Zaleska M, et al: Ribavirin effect on pulmonary function in young infants with respiratory syncytial virus bronchiolitis. *Pediatr Infect Dis J* 1993;12:214-218.

40. Law BJ, Wang EE, MacDonald N, et al: Does ribavirin impact on the hospital course of children with respiratory syncytial virus (RSV) infection? An analysis using the pediatric investiga-

tors collaborative network on infections in Canada (PICNIC) RSV database [abstract]. *Pediatrics* 1997;99:E7.

41. Reassessment of the indications for ribavirin therapy in respiratory syncytial virus infections. American Academy of Pediatrics Committee on Infectious Diseases. *Pediatrics* 1996;97:137-140.

42. Knight V, McClung HW, Wilson SZ, et al: Ribavirin small-particle aerosol treatment of influenza. *Lancet* 1981;2:945-949.

43. Englund JA, Piedra PA, Jefferson LS, et al: High-dose, short-duration ribavirin aerosol therapy in children with suspected respiratory syncytial virus infection. *J Pediatr* 1990;117:313-320.

44. Hall CB, Powell KR, Schnabel KC, et al: Risk of secondary bacterial infection in infants hospitalized with respiratory syncytial virus infection. *J Pediatr* 1988;113:266-271.

45. Glezen WB, Paredes A, Allison JE, et al: Risk of respiratory syncytial virus infection in infants from low-income families in relationship to age, sex, ethnic group, and maternal antibody level. *J Pediatr* 1981;98:708-715.

46. Prince GA, Hemming VG, Horsewood RL, et al: Immuno-prophylaxis and immunotherapy of respiratory syncytial virus infection in the cotton rat. *Virus Res* 1985;3:193-206.

47. Parrot RH, Kim HW, Arrobio JO, et al: Epidemiology of respiratory syncytial virus infection in Washington, DC. II. Infection and disease with respect to age, immunologic status, race, and sex. *Am J Epidemiol* 1973;98:289-300.

48. Hemming VG, Prince GA: Respiratory syncytial virus: babies and antibodies. *Infect Agents Dis* 1992;1:24-32.

49. Hemming VG, Rodriguez WJ, Kim HW, et al: Intravenous immunoglobulin treatment of respiratory syncytial virus infections in infants and young children. *Antimicrob Agents Chemother* 1987;31:1882-1886.

50. Rodriguez WJ, Gruber WC, Groothuis JR, et al: Respiratory syncytial virus immune globulin treatment of RSV lower respiratory tract infection in previously healthy children. *Pediatrics* 1997;100:937-942.

51. Rodriguez WJ, Gruber WC, Welliver RC, et al: Respiratory syncytial virus (RSV) immune globulin intravenous therapy for RSV lower respiratory tract infection in infants and young children at high risk for severe RSV infections: Respiratory Syncytial Virus Immune Globulin Study Group. *Pediatrics* 1997;99:454-461.

52. Taylor G, Stott EJ, Bew M, et al: Monoclonal antibodies protect against respiratory syncytial virus. *Lancet* 1983;2:976.

53. Johnson S, Oliver C, Prince GA, et al: Development of a humanized monoclonal antibody (MEDI-493) with potent in vitro and in vivo activity against respiratory syncytial virus. *J Infect Dis* 1997;176:1215-1224.

54. De Vincenzo JF, Malley R, Ramilo O, et al: Viral concentration in upper and lower respiratory secretions from respiratory syncytial virus (RSV) infected children treated with RSV monoclonal antibody (MEDI-493). *Pediatr Res* 1998;43:144A. Abstract #830.

55. Saez-Llorenz X, Moreno MT, Ramilo O, et al: Phase I/II, double-blind, placebo-controlled, multi-dose escalation trial of a humanized respiratory syncytial virus (RSV) monoclonal antibody (MEDI-493) in children hospitalized with RSV. *Pediatr Res* 1998;43:156A. Abstract # 906.

56. Graham BS, Davis TH, Tang YW: Immunoprophylaxis and immunotherapy of respiratory syncytial virus-infected mice with respiratory syncytial virus-specific immune serum. *Pediatr Res* 1993;34:167-172.

57. Gruber WC, Wilson SZ, Throop BJ, et al: Immunoglobulin administration and ribavirin therapy: efficacy in respiratory syncytial virus infection of the cotton rat. *Pediatr Res* 1987;21:270-274.

58. Prince GA, Porter DD: Treatment of parainfluenza virus type 3 bronchiolitis and pneumonia in a cotton rat model using topical antibody and glucocorticosteroid. *J Infect Dis* 1996;173:598-608.

59. De Vincenzo JP, Leombruno D, Soiffer RJ, et al; Immunotherapy of respiratory syncytial virus pneumonia following bone marrow transplantation. *Bone Marrow Transplant* 1996;17:1051-1056.

60. Bowden RA: Respiratory virus infection after marrow transplant: the Fred Hutchinson Cancer Research Center experience. *Am J Med* 1997;102: 27-30,42-43.

61. Whimbey E, Englund JA, Couch RB: Community respiratory virus infections in immunocompromised patients with cancer. *Am J Med* 1997;102:10-18, 25-26.

62. Whimbey E: *Community Respiratory Viral Infections in the Immunocompetent and Immunocompromised Host.* Tampa, FL, Oncology New Concepts, 1997, pp 4-9.

Chapter **9**

Current Prevention Strategies

Stephen A. Chartrand, MD

Professor and Chairman,
Creighton University School of Medicine,
Omaha, Nebraska

Respiratory syncytial virus (RSV) is now recognized as a major cause of lower respiratory tract infections in children worldwide. Currently, there is no safe and effective vaccine against RSV, and therapy with ribavirin is expensive, cumbersome, and only marginally effective. This chapter reviews the microbiology and immunology of RSV as it is related to prevention strategies. A more detailed discussion of potential RSV vaccines is found in Chapter 10.

Microbiology

The paramyxoviridae family of viruses, which includes the measles virus and the parainfluenza viruses, is the chief cause of respiratory tract infections in humans and other primate species. RSV is the only human pathogen of the paramyxoviridae family in the genus pneumovirus. The RSV genome consists of a single-stranded, negatively coiled RNA segment that encodes for 12 gene products, including the immunologically important F and G glycoproteins common to all members of this family (Figure 1). There are 2 RSV subgroups, A and B, based on the immunoreactivity of the surface G glycoprotein. There is

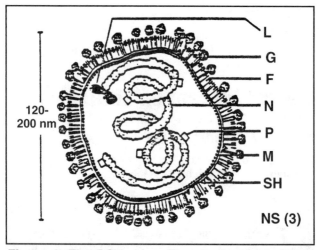

Figure 1: The RSV virion. The single-stranded RNA genome encodes for the G and F surface glycoproteins, which are targets for host-neutralizing antibodies. The G (attachment) glycoprotein attaches to surface receptors on epithelial cells. The F (fusion) glycoprotein mediates viral envelope fusion with host cell membranes, and host cell fusion (syncytia formation).

some evidence that, at least in the United States, group A strains are more virulent than group B, which may partially explain some of the variable severity of annual RSV epidemics.[1] However, a recent study from Denmark found group B strains more virulent, and several studies have observed no difference between the virulence of A and B strains.[2] Because RSV contains only a single strand of RNA, it is less likely to demonstrate genetic variability or reassortment over time, an important fact when developing any type of RSV prophylaxis strategy. If genetic drift or shift occurred regularly with RSV, such as occurs with the segmented genome of the influenza virus, then any prophylactic regimen would lose its effectiveness over time or require continuous modification. Fortunately, immunologically significant alterations in RSV surface antigens occur slowly, if at all.

The surface F and G glycoproteins are the primary targets for host-neutralizing antibody responses. The G glycoprotein directs viral attachment to a specific receptor on the host's respiratory tract epithelial cells. Therefore, if attachment could be prevented by neutralizing the G glycoprotein, infection could be aborted. In fact, convalescent sera from RSV-infected individuals contain high titers of neutralizing anti-G antibody. Unfortunately, there is less than 53% genetic homology for the G glycoprotein among RSV isolates, so any approach directed solely at this antigen will fail to prevent almost half of all infections.[3]

Once the RSV virion has attached itself to the epithelial cell surface, the F glycoprotein mediates fusion of the viral envelope with the cell's lipid membrane. Viral RNA is then injected into the cell's cytoplasm and replication ensues. This fusion function is important in allowing cell-to-cell transmission of RSV along the respiratory tract, resulting in very little cell-free virus that would be susceptible to inhibition by local antibodies. Histologically, this process results in the formation of giant cells (syncytia) in vivo, identical to the in vitro phenomenon. In contrast to the G glycoprotein, the F glycoprotein is highly conserved among all RSV isolates examined to date, worldwide. High titers of anti-F neutralizing antibody are found in convalescent sera, and could prevent initial viral penetration and subsequent spread; thus, the F glycoprotein is a very attractive target for RSV-prevention strategies.

Immune Response to RSV

The role of antibodies in protection against RSV infection was not always clear. RSV infections occur at an early age, when it seems that adequate levels of transplacental antibodies should be present. In fact, very young babies are often the most severely affected, although it is well known that severe bronchiolitis is relatively less common in the first 30 days of life. Moreover, the disastrous experience with the formalin-inactivated RSV vaccine trials in the 1960s led many to believe that anti-RSV antibody was, in fact, deleterious.[4,5] In those trials, children who were immunized with a formalin-inactivated RSV vaccine actually suffered increased pulmonary morbidity and mortality when they acquired natural RSV infection in the next season. At the time, this increased disease severity was thought to be caused by immune complex deposits in the lungs. Today, it is widely thought that an exaggerated T-cell response or imbalance was the true culprit. However, this experience dissuaded researchers from pursuing the role of RSV antibody in prophylaxis for many years.

It was nearly 2 decades later, in 1981, that Glezen et al first demonstrated that high titers of functional (neutralizing) antibody correlated with later-onset and less-severe RSV infection in young, full-term infants,[6] an observation that has been confirmed in subsequent studies.[7,8] Serum-neutralizing antibody responses of both IgG (primarily IgG1) and IgM isotypes occur after infection, but protection is both incomplete and of short duration.[9] Persistence of antibody response (and protection) probably requires reinfection, because RSV is primarily a mucosal-surface pathogen and lacks a viremic phase to expose the organism to the entire array of immune system components. Secretory antibody responses occur predominantly in the IgA isotype after infection and may coincide with termination of viral shedding, but they do not correlate with immunity to reinfection. Correlation with protection is greater with serum than with secretory antibodies.

Patients with defects in cell-mediated immunity (CMI) shed RSV for prolonged periods; this indicates that CMI is important in terminating infection. However, there is some evidence that lymphocyte-transformation responses are greater in severely ill wheezing infants, suggesting that an uncontrolled T-cell response plays a role in severe disease.

Prevention

RSV is easily transmitted via large-droplet aerosol during close contact or by fomites. Virions may survive for up to 45 minutes on clothing or bed sheets and for 6 hours on hard surfaces, such as toys, tabletops, or stethoscopes.[3] Hand-to-eye-or-nose spread is the most common mode of transmission both in the community and in the hospital, and good hand-washing is the most important prevention strategy. For most hospitals, gown and glove isolation is recommended, but if children are assigned to individual rooms, then universal precautions and good hand-washing should suffice. For those in close contact with infectious secretions, masks and protective eyewear should be considered. Whenever possible, nursing personnel should be cohorted to infants with RSV infection and not be simultaneously assigned to high-risk patients. Nurses and other medical staff with suspected upper respiratory RSV infections should not be assigned to high-risk patients, such as premature infants, bone marrow transplant recipients, or other immunosuppressed individuals.

Previously healthy children may shed RSV for 7 to 10 days and immunocompromised patients may shed RSV for weeks, even when treated with ribavirin. Patients with confirmed RSV infection should remain in isolation until cultures test negative. Since most immunocompetent children with acute RSV infection are discharged within 3 to 5 days, they usually remain isolated for the duration of their hospitalization. Immunocompromised hosts should remain isolated until their cultures test negative. RSV antigen-detection tests may remain positive even after cultures come back negative, and should not be used to determine communicability. When infants with community-acquired RSV infection are admitted to the hospital, care should be taken to avoid nosocomial transmission.

Early Preemptive Antiviral Therapy

Currently, the only available antiviral drug for treating RSV is ribavirin, a virustatic nucleoside analogue administered via a small-particle aerosol generator. Therapy with ribavirin is expensive, and its clinical efficacy in established infections is modest at best. Nevertheless, Groothuis et al reasoned that early, aggressive ribavirin treatment in high-risk infants may prevent the development of more severe disease.[10]

In a 3-year, prospective, blinded study, Groothuis et al administered ribavirin to 47 high-risk children < 36 months of age who had laboratory-confirmed RSV infection and mild symptoms for 72 hours. Children were enrolled either at home after manifestation of the first signs of upper respiratory infection or immediately upon admission to the hospital. After 3 days of therapy, there was significant improvement in oxygen saturation in ribavirin-treated patients compared to controls. However, there was no significant difference in respiratory scores or total hospital days between the groups, and treatment failures occurred in similar numbers of patients in both groups. The authors concluded that early ribavirin therapy may help reduce morbidity from RSV infections, but offers no real benefit in preventing hospitalization. Given the high cost of administering the drug and the large number of mildly ill patients that would be treated, early ribavirin therapy is not recommended.

Immune Globulin

Some commercial lots of standard intravenous immunoglobulin (IGIV) may contain substantial levels of neutralizing antibodies to RSV. Large doses of standard IGIV administered to cotton rats and adult monkeys resulted in significant reductions in virus from bronchoalveolar lavage fluid and nasal secretions.[11] These results prompted Hemming et al and Meissner et al to administer selected high-titer lots of commercial IGIV to high-risk infants with acute RSV infection.[12,13] The infusions were well tolerated, produced reductions in nasal virus, and resulted in significant improvements in oxygenation. However, the mean duration of hospitalization was not significantly reduced in these patients vs controls. Groothuis et al safely administered 500 to 750 mg/kg of selected lots of IGIV to high-risk children as prophylaxis.[14] Unequivocal demonstration of efficacy, defined as a reduction in duration of hospital stay, was not observed in these trials, probably because the peak titer of RSV-neutralizing antibody (mean ratio, 1:87) did not reach protection-conferring values (mean ratio, 1:390). Subsequent lots of IGIV that were screened for RSV antibody were found to be lacking in sufficient RSV titers, and trough values after intravenous dosing of such lots were subtherapeutic. Because of the large volume of standard IGIV needed to produce adequate peak and trough anti-RSV levels, this approach has been abandoned.

RSV Intravenous Immunoglobulin (RSV-IGIV, RespiGam™)

The questionable efficacy obtained with standard IGIV provided the impetus to develop an enriched (hyperimmune) RSV globulin, RSV-IGIV (RespiGam™). RSV-IGIV lots for intravenous use were prepared from plasma obtained by plasmapheresis from donors with RSV antibody titers of 3,000 microneutralization units against a stock laboratory strain of RSV.[15] Immunoglobulin suitable for intravenous administration was purified from pooled plasma by the cold ethanol fractionation method and modified in its final steps by using ultrafiltration to minimize aggregation of IgG. RSV-IGIV is approximately 6-fold enriched for neutralizing antibodies (compared with standard commercial IGIV), and was 10 times more potent in reducing pulmonary titers of RSV in cotton rats.[15] RSV-IGIV neutralizes a wide variety of serotype A and B RSV strains in vitro, although titers are generally greater against type A. Beginning in 1989, Groothuis et al conducted a multiyear, randomized, blinded, dose-ranging study of RSV-IGIV in 249 infants and young children with bronchopulmonary dysplasia (BPD), congenital heart disease, or prematurity.[16] Outcome criteria included incidence of RSV upper and lower respiratory tract infection, hospitalization rate, and severity of illness. In the high-dose (750 mg/kg monthly) group, there were fewer lower respiratory tract infections (P=.001), fewer hospitalizations (P=0.02), fewer hospital days (P=0.02), fewer days in the intensive care unit (ICU) (P=0.05), and less use of ribavirin (P=0.05). This study suggested that administration of high doses of RSV-IGIV was safe and effective in preventing lower respiratory tract infections in high-risk infants and young children.

The definitive study with RSV-IGIV was conducted during the 1994-1995 RSV season in 54 centers across the United States.[17] In this double-blind, placebo-controlled trial (PREVENT), 510 children with BPD and/or a history of prematurity were randomized to receive either 750 mg/kg of RSV-IGIV or placebo intravenously every 30 days during RSV season. The primary outcome criterion was hospitalization caused by RSV. Data were also collected about the total days of RSV-related hospital stay, total days of increased oxygen requirement, total days with a moderate or severe lower respiratory tract illness, frequency and duration of ICU stay, and mechanical ventilation. Ninety-five percent of participants completed the protocol, and 85% received a complete course of infusions. The number of children reporting at least 1 adverse event was equal between the 2 treatment groups, as was the severity of these events. Overall, 1.8% of children required interruption of infusion because of problems with fluid volume, and 8.4% required extra diuretics during at least 1 infusion. Children with cyanotic congenital heart disease were more likely to experience adverse events, such as sudden unexplained death associated with cardiac surgery, if they received RSV-IGIV. Various theories, such as hyperviscosity syndrome or hypercoagulable states, have been put forth to explain this observation, but so far, a definitive cause has not been proven. In the meantime, children with cyanotic congenital heart disease should not receive RSV-IGIV.

Compared to the placebo group, the incidence of RSV hospitalization was reduced by 41% in children receiving RSV-IGIV (13.5% vs 8.0%, P=.047). The total number of hospital days, days with increased oxygen requirement, and days with moderate or greater severity of infection scores were all significantly lower in the RSV-IGIV group. Total days in the ICU and mechanical ventilation requirements were low in both groups and not significantly different. The total number of respiratory hospitalizations was also significantly lower in the RSV-IGIV group (27% vs 16%, P=.005). This was probably because RSV-IGIV is a polyclonal product and may contain antibodies against other respiratory pathogens, such as influenza and parainfluenza viruses, and *Streptococcus pneumoniae*. For the same reason, the incidence of acute otitis media was significantly less in a subgroup of 109 children who received RSV-IGIV as part of this study.[18]

Reductions in RSV hospitalizations ranged from 17% to 74% when analyzed by age, gender, and inclusion (ie, prematurity alone, BPD, CHD, etc) categories. Nevertheless, the PREVENT trial was not designed or empowered to detect statistically significant differences in subgroups of the enrollees; therefore, no conclusions could be drawn regarding subgroup efficacy.

Recommendations for the use of RSV-IGIV have been published by a consensus group of experts and the Committee on Infectious Diseases of the American Academy of Pediatrics.[19,20] The recommendations of both groups

Table 1: Indications for the Use of Palivizumab or RSV-IGIV*

- Infants < 2 years old with chronic lung disease (CLD) who are currently receiving or have received medical therapy (eg, oxygen, diuretics, bronchodilators) within 6 months before the RSV season.
- Infants born at 29-32 weeks' gestation with or without CLD, for up to 6 months of age.
- Infants born at 28 weeks' gestation without CLD, for up to 12 months of age.
- Infants born at 32-35 weeks' gestation, when additional risk factors are present. These include underlying neurologic conditions that predispose to respiratory infections, the number of young siblings, daycare attendance, exposure to tobacco smoke, anticipated cardiac surgery, and distance to and availability of hospital care.
- RSV-IGIV is not approved or recommended for infants with congenital heart disease (CHD). However, infants who meet one or both of the first 2 criteria, and who have asymptomatic acyanotic CHD should be considered for prophylaxis.
- Although RSV-IGIV has not been evaluated in randomized clinical trials in immunocompromised patients, children with severe immunodeficiencies may benefit from RSV-IGIV prophylaxis. (The consensus group felt that RSV-IGIV prophylaxis "may be reasonable" for pre-engraftment bone marrow transplant patients during community RSV outbreaks.)
- Infants or children with severe immunodeficiency (eg, SCID or AIDS) may benefit from having RSV-IGIV substituted for routine monthly infusions of γ-globulin. There have not been clinical trials for either RSV-IGIV or palivizumab in this population.

* Adapted from References 19, 20, 28, and 29.

are similar, and are summarized in Table 1. Prophylaxis with RSV-IGIV should be started before the onset of the RSV season and terminated at the end of the RSV season. In most temperate climate areas in North America, the peak season is sometime between November 1st and April 1st, but the actual peak varies from year to year and is unpredictable. Practically, prophylaxis should be started in mid to late October and continued through April 1st. In southern states, the RSV season may begin earlier, and prophylaxis may be required for a longer period. Even if the season peaks early, prophylaxis should be continued, because multiple RSV episodes during the same season are well documented and may be severe in high-risk infants.

Infants receiving RSV-IGIV prophylaxis should not receive live-virus vaccines (eg, measles, mumps, rubella, and varicella) for 9 months after the last RSV-IGIV dose and should have their vaccination repeated after that time because of possible interference with the immune response. All other routine childhood vaccines (including oral poliovirus, if needed) may be given without regard to RSV-IGIV dosing.

In the PREVENT trial, there was a significant reduction in non-RSV respiratory hospitalizations in infants who received RSV-IGIV. It appears that the lots of RSV-IGIV administered in the study contained significant levels of antibody against strains of non-RSV respiratory viruses that were circulating during the 1994-1995 season. However, this may not always be the case, since the antiviral spectrum of RSV-IGIV will always reflect the shared infectious experiences of the donors. When practitioners deliberate whether to administer RSV-IGIV or palivizumab, they should not presume that RSV-IGIV will always provide additional protection against new influenza strains.

Despite the proven efficacy of RSV-IGIV in preventing RSV hospitalizations, monthly infusions are cumber-

Table 2: Drawbacks to RSV-IGIV Prophylaxis
• Need for intravenous access
• Potential for adverse effects
-infusion-related events
-excess fluid volume
-transmission of blood-borne pathogens
• Interference with live-virus vaccines
• Time and resource commitments
• May be stressful for parents
• Expensive

some, expensive, time consuming, and stressful for parents (Table 2). Even with a restricted, well-defined donor pool and strict manufacturing quality-control measures, there is always the remote possibility of blood-borne pathogen transmission.

Anti-RSV Monoclonal Antibody (Palivizumab, Synagis™)

One approach to improve the specific activity of anti-RSV immunoglobulin is to develop a highly potent RSV-neutralizing monoclonal antibody (MAb). MAbs should be human or humanized in order to retain favorable pharmacokinetics and avoid generating a human antimouse antibody response, since repeat dosing is required throughout the RSV season. In 1997, researchers at MedImmune, Inc. developed a humanized murine monoclonal antibody, palivizumab (Synagis™), that recognizes a conserved neutralizing epitope ('A' region) on the F glycoprotein of RSV (Figure 2).[21] The generic name, palivizumab, is derived from 'pali' meaning 'palliation,' 'viz' for 'virus,' 'u' for

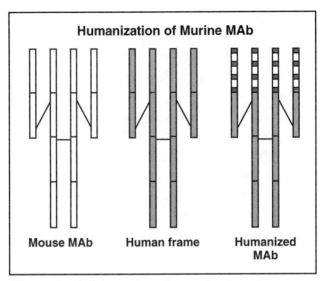

Figure 2: *Palivizumab, a humanized murine mono-clonal antibody (MAb) to RSV. Using recombinant techniques, F glycoprotein epitope binding sites are transferred from a murine MAb into the backbone of a human IgG1 molecule. The final product, palivizumab, retains the immunologic specificity and activity of the murine antibody, but is > 90% human in origin.*

'humanized,' and 'mab' for monoclonal antibody. The original murine antibody was humanized by inserting the complementary regions from an F glycoprotein-specific neutralizing murine MAb into a human IgG1 framework.[22] The grafted binding sites contain no murine antigenic elements, so the final MAb is, immunologically, virtually indistinguishable from a complete human IgG1 antibody. Palivizumab is broadly reactive against all subtype A and B RSV strains tested to date, worldwide. It is approximately 50 to 100 times more active than RSV-IGIV in vitro and in the cotton rat model. In preliminary studies, palivizumab was safe and well tolerated in high-risk infants, who were administered 15 mg/kg intravenously every 30 days (Table 3).[23] These doses maintained serum concentrations of > 40 mg/L that were associated with a 99% RSV reduction in the cotton rat model. This established 40 mg/L as the target level for prophylaxis. The pharmacokinetic profile of palivizumab is virtually identical when given intravenously or intramuscularly (IM).[24]

The definitive palivizumab study was a randomized, double-blind, placebo-controlled trial conducted at 139 centers in the United States, the United Kingdom, and Canada during the 1996-1997 RSV season.[25] In this trial, known as the IMpact study, children were eligible if they were either: 1) 35 weeks' gestation or less and 6 months of age or younger; or 2) 24 months of age or younger, and had a clinical diagnosis of BPD requiring ongoing medical treatment (ie, supplemental oxygen, steroids, bronchodilators, or diuretics within the past 6 months). A total of

1,502 patients were randomized 2:1 to receive either palivizumab at 15 mg/kg IM every 30 days or placebo, during the RSV season. Overall, 94% of the placebo group and 92% of the palivizumab group received all 5 injections between November and March. Mean trough serum concentrations 30 days after palivizumab injection ranged from 37 to 72 mg/L, with some accumulation after repeated doses. Monthly prophylaxis was associated with a 55% (95% CI = 38, 72%) reduction in RSV hospitalizations (P=.00004). Significant reductions were observed both in children with BPD (39%, P=.038) and without BPD (78%, P <.001). In contrast to the PREVENT study, in which subgroup analysis was not possible, the sample size in the IMpact trial (1,002 patients) was large enough to detect significant reductions in RSV hospitalizations in several subgroups (Figure 3). Children randomized to receive palivizumab had significantly fewer total days of RSV hospitalization, fewer days with increased oxygen needs, and fewer days with a lower respiratory infection score of 3 or more (moderate-to-severe illness). The incidence of ICU admissions was low for both groups, but was less in the palivizumab group (1.3% vs 3.9%, P=.026). There was no difference in the total number of ICU days or requirement for mechanical ventilation. Palivizumab recipients had significant reductions in the incidence and total days of all hospitalizations, and the incidence and total days of respiratory hospitalizations. These differences were attributable to the observed reduction in RSV hospitalizations, because no significant differences were observed in the incidence or total days of hospitalization unrelated to RSV. In contrast to the findings in the PREVENT study, there was no reduction in the incidence of acute otitis media in palivizumab recipients. There was no significant difference in the spectrum or frequency of adverse events between the 2 groups. Antimurine antibodies were rarely detected in either group, nor did they increase in frequency with subsequent dosing.

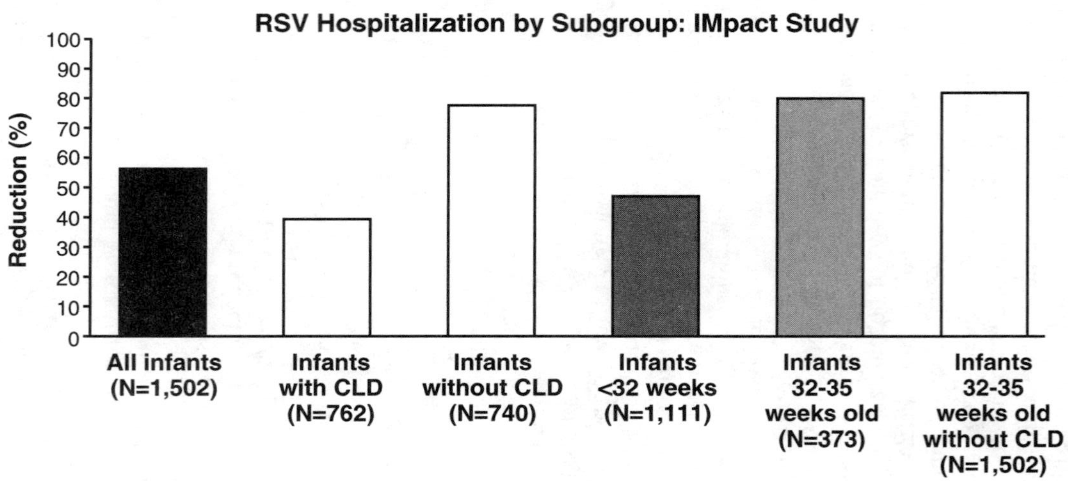
RSV Hospitalization by Subgroup: IMpact Study
Reduction (%)
100
90
80
70
60
50
40
30
20
10
0
All infants (N=1,502)
Infants with CLD (N=762)
Infants without CLD (N=740)
Infants <32 weeks (N=1,111)
Infants 32-35 weeks old (N=373)
Infants 32-35 weeks old without CLD (N=1,502)

The IMpact Study Group, 1998.

Figure 3: *Subgroup analysis of palivizumab: IMpact study.*

The results from the PREVENT and IMpact studies cannot be directly compared, because these 2 investigations were carried out with different populations in different years. Nevertheless, given the enhanced in vitro activity of palivizumab, one might question why a greater reduction in RSV hospitalization rates was not seen in all groups. For example, palivizumab was more effective in reducing hospitalizations in infants with prematurity alone, compared to those with chronic lung disease (CLD), such as BPD. This makes sense, because those with severe BPD are more fragile, and perhaps even mild RSV disease is poorly tolerated. Nevertheless, this finding is almost the opposite of the findings in the PREVENT study, where efficacy appeared better in those with CLD. Canfield and Simoes have postulated that, in premature infants, palivizumab replaced only the deficient anti-RSV antibodies, whereas, because of the large dose (750 mg/kg), RSV-IGIV also had a significant anti-inflammatory effect in the lung.[26]

Some experts have expressed concern that resistance in the form of 'escape mutants' might occur with widespread use of palivizumab, since in vitro resistance has occurred with other MAbs. Escape mutants alter surface proteins that could change the configuration of the antigenic site, shielding the binding site from the antibody. However, Branco et al recently reported an evaluation of more than 500 RSV isolates collected worldwide during the past 10 years.[27] Palivizumab was able to bind to all these strains, suggesting that resistance to palivizumab, at least for now, does not exist.

The Committee on Infectious Diseases and the Committee on Fetus and Newborn of the American Academy of Pediatrics (AAP), and a separate expert consensus group, have published recommendations for the use of palivizumab.[28,29] These recommendations are similar to those published earlier for the use of RSV-IGIV in high-risk infants. However, the palivizumab guidelines have been broadened to include specified infants between 32 and 35 weeks' gestational age. To maximize relative benefit and cost effectiveness, the AAP now recommends that only those infants with specific additional risk factors be considered for prophylaxis (Table 1). Given the 80% reduction in RSV hospitalization in the 32- to 35-weeks gestational age group in the phase III IMpact trial, one may question why any part of this group is still excluded. It is important that additional studies be performed of RSV hospitalization in the 32- to 35-weeks gestational age group. If RSV rehospitalization rates are found to be low in this group, benefits of prophylaxis might be less than anticipated and the present guidelines may need to be reviewed.

Palivizumab was licensed in the United States in 1998 and in Europe in 1999 under the trade name of Synagis™ ('Syn' = syncytial, 'agis' = shield [Greek]). Postlicensure data on the efficacy of palivizumab through the first 2 years are now available. Such information is important because some critics have claimed that much of the reduction in RSV admissions came from increased parent education and attention that study patients received from research personnel, and therefore, would not be reproducible in the real-world setting. In the Outcomes study, a retrospective chart review was conducted of 1,839 high-risk infants in 9 centers across the United States during the 1998-1999 and 1999-2000 RSV seasons. The readmission rate for proven RSV infection was 2.3%, compared to 4.8% seen during the IMpact study.[30] Preliminary unpublished results for the 1999-2000 Outcomes study season show a similar readmission rate of only 2.4% (MedImmune, Inc., personal communication, August 2000). In an open-label study of 565 high-risk infants in Europe (the Expanded Access study), researchers found a readmission rate of only 2.1% caused by RSV infections (MedImmune, Inc., personal communication, August 2000). Although these were not controlled trials, the data suggest that real-world experience with palivizumab is comparable to the research findings, at least in the first 2 years postlicensure.

Education

No RSV-prevention program would be complete or appropriate without a heavy emphasis on preventive education of hospital staff and families. During the RSV season, a health-care worker education program should be instituted on the importance of good hand-washing, cohorting of potentially RSV-infected infants, and restricting workers with symptoms of upper respiratory tract infection from contact with high-risk individuals (premature infants, immunocompromised hosts, patients with chronic lung disease, etc). Parents of NICU graduates should be cautioned against passive smoke exposure, crowding, placing high-risk infants into large day-care centers during RSV season, and they should be advised to limit contact with individuals exhibiting obvious signs of upper respiratory tract infection. Physicians responsible for high-risk infants should keep a list of prophylaxis candidates and begin educating parents about the hazards of RSV before the child is discharged from the ICU. As in any health-care maintenance program, providers should reinforce this information at each follow-up visit. Telephone calls or postcards to providers and parents of all high-risk infants before the start of RSV season, reminding them of the need for prophylaxis (just as many offices do for routine immunizations) might be considered. Finally, insurers should be contacted well in advance of the RSV season to ensure prophylaxis coverage, including arrangements for administration.

Summary

Comprehensive RSV-prevention programs should be implemented for all high-risk infants, including education to minimize RSV exposure; reasonable infection control measures, especially good hand-washing; and monthly prophylaxis with either palivizumab or RSV-IGIV for selected high-risk infants during the RSV season. For most children, with the possible exception of immunosuppressed infants currently receiving γ-globulin infusions or those with severely compromised chronic lung disease,[28] the ease of administration and decreased cost of palivizumab make it the preferred option over RSV-IGIV.

References

1.　Walsh EE, McConnochie KI, Long CE, et al: Severity of respiratory syncytial virus infection is related to virus strain. *J Infect Dis* 1997;175:814-820.

2.　Hornsleth A, Klug B, Nir M, et al: Severity of respiratory syncytial virus disease related to type and genotype of virus and to cytokine values in nasopharyngeal secretions. *Pediatr Infect Dis J* 1998;17:1114-1121.

3.　Ruuskanen O, Ogra PL: Respiratory syncytial virus. *Curr Prob Pediatr* 1993;8:50-79.

4.　Kapikian AZ, Mitchell RH, Chanock RM, et al: An epidemiologic study of altered clinical reactivity to respiratory syncytial (RS) virus infection in children previously vaccinated with an inactivated RS virus vaccine. *Am J Epidemiol* 1969;89:405-421.

5.　Kim HW, Canchola JG, Brandt CD, et al: Respiratory syncytial virus disease in infants despite prior administration of antigenic inactivated vaccine. *Am J Epidemiol* 1969;89:422-434.

6.　Glezen WP, Paredes A, Allison J, et al: Risk of respiratory syncytial virus infection for infants from low-income families in relationship to age, sex, ethnic group, and maternal antibody level. *J Pediatr* 1981;98;708-715.

7.　Glezen WP, Taber LH, Frank AL, et al: Risk of primary infection and reinfection with respiratory syncytial virus. *Am J Dis Child* 1986;140:543-546.

8.　Wang EE, Law BJ, Robinson, JL, et al: PICNIC (Pediatric Investigators Collaborative Network on Infections in Canada) study of the role of age and respiratory syncytial virus microneutralizing antibody on RSV illness in patients with underlying heart or lung disease. *Pediatrics* 1997;99:E9.

9.　Hall CB, Walsh EE, Long CE, et al: Immunity to and frequency of reinfection with respiratory syncytial virus. *J Infect Dis* 1991;163:693-698.

10. Groothuis JR, Woodin KA, Katz R, et al: Early ribavirin treatment of respiratory syncytial virus infection in high-risk children. *J Pediatr* 1990;117:792-798.

11. Hemming VG, Prince GA, Groothuis JR, et al: Hyperimmune globulins in prevention and treatment of respiratory syncytial virus infections. *Clin Microbiol Rev* 1995;8:22-33.

12. Hemming VG, Rodriguez W, Kim HW, et al: Intravenous immunoglobulin treatment of respiratory syncytial virus infections in infants and young children. *Antimicrob Agents Chemother* 1987;31:1882-1886.

13. Meissner HC, Fulton DR, Groothuis JR, et al: Controlled trial to evaluate protection of high-risk infants against respiratory syncytial virus disease by using standard intravenous immune globulin. *Antimicrob Agents Chemother* 1993;37:1655-1658.

14. Groothuis JR, Levin MJ, Rodriguez W, et al: Use of intravenous gamma globulin to passively immunize high-risk children against respiratory syncytial virus: safety and pharmacokinetics. The RSVIG Study Group. *Antimicrob Agents Chemother* 1991;35:1469-1473.

15. Siber GR, Leombruno D, Leszczynski J, et al: Comparison of antibody concentrations and protective activity of respiratory syncytial virus immune globulin and conventional immune globulin. *J Infect Dis* 1994;169:1368-1373.

16. Groothuis JR, Simoes EA, Levin MJ, et al: Prophylactic administration fo respiratory syncytial virus immune globulin to high-risk infants and young children. The Respiratory Syncytial Virus Immune Globulin Study Group. *N Engl J Med* 1993;329:1524-1530.

17. Reduction of respiratory syncytial virus hospitalization among premature infants and infants with bronchopulmonary dysplasia using respiratory syncytial virus immune globulin prophylaxis. The PREVENT Study Group. *Pediatrics* 1997;99:93-99.

18. Simoes EA, Groothuis JR, Tristram DA, et al: Respiratory syncytial virus-enriched globulin for the prevention of acute otitis media in high-risk children. *J Pediatr* 1996;129:214-219.

19. Meissner HC, Welliver RC, Chartrand SA, et al: Prevention of respiratory syncytial virus infection in high-risk infants: consensus opinion on the role of immunoprophylaxis with respiratory syncytial virus hyperimmune globulin. *Pediatr Infect Dis J* 1996;15:1059-1068.

20.   Respiratory syncytial virus immune globulin intravenous: indications for use. American Academy of Pediatrics Committee on Infectious Diseases, Committee on Fetus and Newborn. *Pediatrics* 1997; 99:645-650.

21.   Johnson S, Oliver C, Prince GA, et al: Development of a humanized monoclonal antibody (MEDI-493) with potent in vitro and in vivo activity against respiratory syncytial virus. *J Infect Dis* 1997;176:1215-1224.

22.   Beeler JA, van Wyke Coelingh K: Neutralization epitopes of the F glycoprotein of respiratory syncytial virus: effect of mutation upon fusion function. *J Virol* 1989;63:2941-2950.

23.   Subramanian KN, Weisman LE, Rhodes T, et al: Safety, tolerance and pharmacokinetics of a humanized monoclonal antibody to respiratory syncytial virus in premature infants and infants with bronchopulmonary dysplasia. MEDI493 Study Group. *Pediatr Infect Dis J* 1998;17:110-115.

24. Saez-Llorens X, Castano E, Sanchez P, et al: Phase I/II, open-label multi-dose escalation trial of a humanized respiratory syncytial virus (RSV) monoclonal antibody (MEDI-493) administered intramuscularly (IM) in high-risk children. Presented at the Interscience Conference on Antimicrobial Agents and Chemotherapy; September-October 1997; Toronto, Canada. Abstract H89.

25.   Palivizumab, a humanized respiratory syncytial virus monoclonal antibody, reduces hospitalization from respiratory syncytial virus infection in high-risk infants. The IMpact-RSV Study Group. *Pediatrics* 1998;102:531-537.

26.   Canfield SD, Simoes EA: Prevention of respiratory syncytial virus (RSV) infection: RSV immune globulin intravenous and palivizumab. American Academy of Pediatrics. *Pediatr Ann* 1999;28:507-514.

27.   Branco L, Barren P, Gross R, et al: Development of a broadly reactive humanized monoclonal antibody for the prevention of severe lower respiratory tract disease caused by respiratory virus. Presented at the Euro-Pediatric Society of Infectious Diseases; May 1999; Crete, Greece.

28.   Prevention of respiratory syncytial virus infections: indications for the use of palivizumab and update on the use of RSV-IGIV. American Academy of Pediatrics, Committee on Infectious Diseases. Committee on Fetus and Newborn. *Pediatrics* 1998;102:1211-1216.

29.   Meissner HC, Welliver RC, Chartrand SA, et al: Immunoprophylaxis with palivizumab, humanized respiratory syncytial virus monoclonal antibody, for prevention of respiratory syncytial virus infection in high-risk infants: a consensus opinion. *Pediatr Infect Dis J* 1999;18:223-231.

30. Sorrentino M, Albin C, Carlin D, et al: Effectiveness of Synagis™ (palivizumab): evaluation of outcomes from the 1998-99 RSV season. *Pediatr Infect Dis J*. In press.

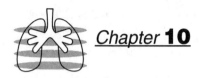

Chapter 10

Future Prevention Strategies

James E. Crowe, Jr, MD

Assistant Professor of Pediatrics
and Microbiology, and Immunology,
Division of Pediatric Infectious Diseases,
Vanderbilt University Medical Center,
Nashville, Tennessee

Janet A. Englund, MD

Associate Professor of Pediatrics,
Division of Pediatric Infectious Diseases,
University of Chicago Hospitals,
Chicago, Illinois

Immunization is likely to be the key to preventing respiratory syncytial virus (RSV) disease. Vaccines are the most likely agents to provide cost-effective protection to the large number of people at risk for RSV disease. However, population groups such as the very young, the immunosuppressed, and the fragile elderly may not be candidates for active immunization, but still must be considered at high risk for serious sequelae from RSV disease. Other strategies, including passive immunization by the use of exogenously administered monoclonal antibodies, may be useful approaches for those unable to mount an active antibody response. The prevention of RSV disease on a widespread basis may ultimately involve several population-based strategies.

Obstacles to Developing RSV Vaccines

Although RSV vaccine development began more than 30 years ago, there is still no licensed RSV vaccine available today. The development and testing processes of vaccine candidates have been hindered by a number of significant obstacles (Table 1). For example, definitive preclinical testing of vaccine candidates is inhibited by the lack of an ideal animal model. Various mouse strains have been studied because of the wealth of immunologic reagents available for these animals, yet the mouse is only a semipermissive host for RSV replication.[1,2] Cotton rats are more susceptible to infection,[3] but the animal's high body temperature and the lack of immunologic reagents significantly limit the systematic study of vaccine candidates. Nonhuman primate studies in animals such as African and Caribbean Green monkeys and chimpanzees have yielded important preclinical results that correlate with data from human trials,[4,5] but even these animals are not as permissive to RSV infection as human infants. Definitive studies of the safety, stability, immunogenicity, and protective efficacy of RSV vaccine candidates can only be carried out in humans. Furthermore, the age-dependent development of immunity and lung growth in humans also ensures that evaluations of potential vaccine products must be carried out carefully and sequentially, starting with adults, progressing to seropositive children and infants, and finally, in seronegative or RSV-naive children and infants.[4,6] This strategy may prove to be successful but requires substantial clinical effort, expertise, and expense.

Only a single serotype of RSV exists, although field isolates exhibit an antigenic dimorphism. Isolates are characterized as belonging to 1 of 2 subgroups, designated A and B, based on reciprocal cross-neutralization studies and genetic analysis.[7,8] Antigenic variation is not required for reinfection by RSV in any particular individual, but the

Table 1: Obstacles to RSV Vaccine Development

- No perfect animal model
- Two antigenic subgroups
- Young age of primary vaccine target population
  - safety concerns in neonates
  - immunologic immaturity
  - possible interactions with other infant vaccines
- Multiple target populations
  - premature, lung disease, cardiac disease
  - immunocompromised
  - asthmatics
  - adults with chronic obstructive pulmonary disease
  - elderly
- Maternal antibodies inhibit immune responses in the target population
- Disease occurs at the portal of entry (the respiratory mucosa)
- Short-lived nature of mucosal immunity to respiratory viruses
- Incomplete immunity to RSV induced by natural infection
- History of vaccine-associated enhanced diseases following FI-RSV

variation may contribute to the high reinfection rate in the population. Therefore, developing a bivalent subgroup A and B vaccine may be required to provide optimal protection against natural infection. Multivalent vaccines are already in widespread use for the prevention of other respiratory diseases, such as influenza.[9] The necessity for coverage of the 2 antigenic RSV subgroups further complicates the development of RSV vaccines.

Another complicating factor in the development of RSV vaccines is that target populations for immunization vary widely with regard to immunologic maturity, experience with previous RSV infection, airway size, and physiology. The vast majority of RSV-related hospitalizations occur in very young infants who are RSV-naive, but possess varied levels of maternally acquired serum antibodies and who have no identifiable risk factors for severe disease.[10,11] Therefore, the principal target population for immunization is normal infants in the first month(s) of life. Other at-risk populations include premature infants and patients with congenital heart disease or chronic lung disease (especially bronchopulmonary dysplasia).[12] Such high-risk patients may continue to have an increased risk of severe RSV disease in the first years of life despite previous naturally acquired RSV infection. Another target population is the elderly,[13] who may have already experienced RSV infection many times in life. One vaccine candidate or strategy may not be optimal for each of these target populations. Indeed, it has already been shown that the same live-attenuated viruses that are not infectious or immunogenic in adults or older children (ie, are overattenuated) may cause disease in the youngest infants (ie, are insufficiently attenuated).[4]

Immunization of the principal target group, the neonate, may be difficult, because of the extreme young age at which protection is required to prevent serious disease. Since the peak incidence of hospitalization in young infants is during the first 2 months of life, induction of adequate immunity will require very early immunization. Furthermore, neonates exhibit a significant immunologic immaturity that may dictate the use of a multidose vaccine strategy ('prime-boost') that will need to be delivered in the first months of life. Safety concerns can be formidable at this age. Active immunization with new RSV vaccines may interfere or interact with the standard vaccines in the current pediatric schedule, many of which are given at 1 or 2 months of age. Furthermore, passively acquired antibodies, such as maternal antibodies, may inhibit the primary immune response of infants to infection or immunization. Although transplacentally acquired antibodies against RSV may protect the infant for the first few weeks or months of life, such antibodies also have the potential to inhibit both serum and secretory antibody responses to immunization. This phenomenon has been observed in epidemiologic studies of wild-type virus infection,[10,14] in experimental infections with live-attenuated vaccine candidates,[4] and in animal model systems such as rodents and primates.[15,16]

Unlike systemic viral infections that initially enter via the respiratory tract and then disseminate, such as measles or varicella zoster virus infection, RSV does not produce a viremia before severe disease. RSV infection and disease occur at the site of entry, namely, the respiratory mucosa. Therefore, in contrast to the licensed viral vaccines, such as the live-attenuated measles or varicella zoster virus vaccines, induction of RSV immunity that is limited to the serum may not be optimal to protect against the most severe clinical diseases associated with RSV. Although clinical efficacy based on adequate levels of serum-neutralizing antibodies has been demonstrated using passive immunization of RSV-specific antibodies,[17,18] maintenance of sterilizing RSV immunity against reinfection at the mucosal surface over the long term after active immunization may not be physiologic or even feasible.

Another problem in the development of an RSV vaccine is the debate over the ultimate purpose of the vaccine. Is the goal to prevent infection, or to prevent disease? The short-lived and incomplete nature of mucosal immunity to viruses suggests that complete immunity against infection may not be a realistic goal for a vaccine strategy. For example, adults with recent RSV infection can be reinfected in the upper respiratory tract multiple times in serial fashion with the same virus suspension.[19]

Ultimately, protection against lower respiratory tract disease during RSV infection appears to be a more feasible goal, since naturally acquired wild-type virus infection of infants appears to provide protection against lower respiratory tract disease.[20,21] This goal, however, contrasts with standard concepts of licensed vaccines, such as the successful conjugate bacterial vaccines against *Haemophilus influenzae* type b and *Streptococcus pneumoniae*. The concept of preventing disease while not necessarily preventing infection necessitates careful design of endpoints for evaluating clinical vaccine field trials.

Finally, the complications of the formalin-inactivated RSV (FI-RSV) vaccine studies in the 1960s have hindered rapid development and testing of RSV vaccine candidates (Chapter 2). In those studies, patients who received FI-RSV immunization suffered much higher rates of severe lower respiratory tract disease.[22,23] Much effort has been expended to define the immune mechanisms underlying the enhanced immunopathology induced by FI-RSV. The testing of RSV subunit vaccines has been particularly complicated by the finding of enhanced histopathology in rodent models.[24] Although nonreplicating antigens may not be the appropriate vaccine candidates for RSV-naive infants, the use of these vaccines as booster immunizations has been considered for previously infected high-risk children,[25,26] for the elderly,[27] and for maternal immunization.[28]

Thus, RSV candidate vaccines face many obstacles. A successful immunization strategy may require distinct approaches directed at different populations. An ideal vaccine candidate could be a genetically stable, multiple-dose bivalent vaccine that could be started in the first weeks of life to stimulate immunity in the presence of maternal antibodies, without inducing enhanced immunopathology. Innovative strategies, such as maternal immunization and passive immunization with monoclonal antibodies, and combinations of these strategies with live-attenuated vaccines, also need to be considered. Finally, improvements in a passively administered antibody may be useful for those individuals unable to mount an effective immune response to active immunization.

RSV Immunity as Related to Vaccination

Immune responses to RSV (reviewed in Chapter 6) are complex and not yet completely understood. Nevertheless, the significant factors that mediate resolution of acute disease and resistance to reinfection have been described. Cytolytic T-lymphocytes (CTLs) are likely to be the principal mediators in resolving acute infection.[29] CTL levels peak at the time that viral clearance is observed during primary infection in experimental animals. Animals and humans lacking T-cells exhibit prolonged RSV shedding.[30,31] CTLs probably do not contribute significantly to protection against reinfection under normal circumstances because the CTL response is short-lived. CTL precursors certainly persist in the host, but activated CTLs are not detected at significant levels several weeks following infection or immunization.[32]

Antibodies are the principal mediators of resisting RSV reinfection. Both secretory and serum antibodies appear to protect against RSV disease and infection.[19,33] Serum RSV IgG antibodies, when present at high levels, protect the lower respiratory tract against infection, but have little impact on upper respiratory tract virus replication.[34] In the upper tract, local antibodies, including secretory IgA, appear to play a major role in protection. Interestingly, the IgAs induced by infection or immunization do not appear to neutralize virus in classical in vitro virus neutralization assays,[6,35] but correlate strongly with protection of the upper respiratory tract,[36] suggesting protection by novel mechanisms. Protective antibodies are directed to the fusion (F) and attachment (G) surface glycoproteins, and emphasis has been placed on studying the response to these proteins. Numerous assays have been developed to describe the quality and quantity of RSV antibodies induced by immunization, and to differentiate responses to wild-type virus infection from vaccine-induced responses.[37] It appears that the majority of antibodies induced by infection that bind to RSV F or G proteins do not neutralize in vitro or protect in vivo.[38] Subsets of antibodies neutralize virus, and some of these antibodies also inhibit virus fusion in vitro. Such neutralizing antibodies appear to be the key to protection against reinfection. Thus, the quality of the immune response to immunization can be characterized by the level of neutralizing antibodies and by the ratio of neutralizing-to-binding antibody levels.

Vaccine Development: Types of Vaccines

Formalin-inactivated RSV (FI-RSV) vaccine trials. Clinical trials conducted in the 1960s using an inactivated RSV preparation were terminated when severe adverse events occurred. Although this strategy is no longer being pursued, understanding the pathogenesis of enhanced disease is essential to future vaccine efforts. The original rationale for using inactivated vaccine was that nonreplicating antigens were thought to carry little risk of reactogenicity, and that inactivated vaccines for other mucosally acquired viruses, such as polio virus and influenza virus, were historically safe and effective. During the trials, the vaccine was prepared from RSV-infected cells that were fixed with formalin and concentrated by ultracentrifugation and alum precipitation, and then administered in multiple doses to infants <7 months of age. Upon subsequent wild-type virus infection, infants were not protected against RSV infection and suffered much higher rates of severe lower respiratory tract disease than did control subjects.

Since those FI-RSV trials, many investigators have sought to define the mechanism for this enhanced disease using some of the original clinical materials or with animal models, principally rodents. Although we recognize that rodents are not ideal for studying RSV infection because of the semipermissive nature of the infection in these hosts, the broad array of available immunologic manipulations has allowed for the construction of reasonable hypotheses about the nature of the enhanced disease. Vaccinees exhibited an altered serum-neutralizing to binding-antibody ratio, suggesting that formalin treatment destroyed or altered the protective neutralizing antigenic sites in the immunizing virus preparation.[39] In animal models, experimental FI-RSV preparations can also prime for a Th2-like cytokine response in the lungs that, upon subsequent infection, is associated with lymphocytic and eosinophilic infiltration without virus-clearing CD8+ CTLs.[24] FI-RSV likely primed for increased immune-mediated airway inflammation without inducing a protective response. Preclinical evaluation of inactivated vaccine candidates must address this potential serious complication.

Live-virus vaccines. Much progress has been made in the development and evaluation of live-attenuated vaccine candidates[39,40] (Table 2). The rationale for this approach is that live-virus infection of the nasopharynx induces a balanced immune response similar to that induced by natural infection, and therefore, is unlikely to induce enhanced disease, such as that associated with FI-RSV. Indeed, enhanced disease has not been observed on subsequent infection following wild-type virus infection or experimental live-virus immunization. Additional advantages of the live-attenuated virus approach are that topical infection induces both secretory and serum antibodies, and can infect subjects even in the presence of passively acquired antibodies, such as maternal antibodies.[6] The initial development of live-attenuated vaccines was based on cell culture manipulations in the laboratory that isolated mutant viruses exhibiting an in vitro phenotype that was correlated with attenuation in vivo. These efforts were similar to those used successfully by Sabin and others to identify the live-attenuated poliovirus vac-

Table 2: Vaccine Approaches to RSV Prevention

Vaccine Type	Example	Reference
Live-attenuated biologically derived	*cpts* 248/404	4
Live-attenuated genetically engineered		41
Vector-delivered	vaccinia virus-F or G	42
	modified vaccinia virus – Ankara	43
	recombinant adenovirus	44
Subunit vaccines	purified fusion protein (PFP-1 and PFP-2)	45
	baculovirus-derived FG chimera	46
	bacterial-derived BB2Gna	47
DNA vaccines	plasmids containing F or G cDNA	48
Peptide vaccines	protective epitopes	49
Animal viruses	bovine-RSV	50

cines. For example, RSV mutant viruses that were cold-passaged (*cp*) or temperature-sensitive (*ts*, ie, grow well at the permissive temperatures of the nasopharynx but not at the higher temperatures of the lungs) were developed and tested in adults, children, and infants.[30] Such viruses were found to be attenuated, infectious, and immunogenic in older infants. However, these early vaccine candidate strains suffered from a low level of loss of the in vitro phenotype during virus shedding in human vaccinees. The clinical significance of this genetic instability was not fully understood, but testing of live-attenuated viruses was discontinued for a number of years as other strategies were explored. Clearly, it is desirable to achieve a high level of genetic stability of the attenuating mutations in a vaccine candidate. Parallel efforts to generate other live-attenuated respiratory virus vaccine candidates have demonstrated that attenuated RNA viruses can be identified that exhibit a high level of genetic stability in humans. Such stability has been demonstrated, for example, in cold-adapted influenza virus vaccines and the parainfluenza virus type 3 (PIV-3) *cp*-45 vaccine candidate.[9,51] The key to the stability of these viruses appears to be the presence of multiple attenuating mutations that are under different types of selective pressure to revert. The influenza and PIV-3 candidate vaccine viruses possess both *ts* and host-range attenuating mutations.

Recently, efforts were renewed to generate live-attenuated RSV vaccine candidates that possess multiple attenuating mutations.[40] Starting with the previously tested host-range mutant *cp*-RSV and introducing a series of multiple *ts* mutations by chemical mutagenesis has resulted in promising vaccine candidates. Viruses that possess the *cp*-RSV attenuating mutations and at least 2 *ts* mutations were found to be highly attenuated and genetically stable in rodents, chimpanzees, and humans, including seronegative infants. At least 4 such mutants have been examined to date in phase I clinical trials in seronegative infants.[4,16] Current efforts center on identifying vaccine candidates that are sufficiently attenuated and immunogenic in the very youngest infants (birth to 2 months).

Live vaccines derived via genetic engineering. In the 1990s, scientists at the National Institutes of Health developed technologies that enabled the generation of live

RSV viruses from plasmid DNA copies (cDNA) of the virus genome.[52] This work has led to development of site-directed mutations in viruses and, thus, the evolution of logical candidate vaccines. First, the genetic basis of attenuation of many of the biologically derived vaccine candidates was determined by nucleotide sequence analysis of cDNA. The *ts* phenotype of these mutants was encoded, in most cases, by single nucleotide changes in open-reading frames or in virus-regulatory regions, such as the gene-start region.[53,54] Subsequently, multiple mutations from separate biologically derived *ts* mutants have been combined into novel viruses that are created in the laboratory from cDNA copies that specify a combination of mutations. Novel mutations, such as deletion of the entire SH, N51, or NS2 gene, have also been introduced.[55] Such viruses exhibit increased levels of attenuation and genetic stability in preclinical models. New constructs, including chimeric viruses with genes encoding proteins from different RSV subtypes, or with genes both deleted and re-arranged within a single strain, are being investigated. It is likely that an appropriately attenuated, genetically stable virus for both subgroups A and B will be generated using these techniques and evaluated in larger clinical studies.

Virus vector delivery systems. Live-virus vectors that encode and express RSV F and G genes have been explored in preclinical models, principally the vaccinia virus and adenovirus.[44,56] Vaccinia viruses that express F (vac-F) or G (vac-G) were generated and found to be immunogenic and protective in rodents. Intradermal immunization with these vaccine candidates was less immunogenic in chimpanzees, and did not protect the lower respiratory tract of these animals against wild-type RSV challenge. The use of vaccinia virus vectors in infants faces significant safety concerns as well, and such vaccines are unlikely to progress to clinical trials. Newer poxvirus vectors expressing RSV proteins that do not produce infectious virus progeny in humans could be considered for use in humans.[43] The evaluation of adenovirus recombinant viruses in large mammals failed to induce adequate levels of protection against RSV.

Subunit vaccines. Protective antibodies against RSV are directed to the F and G proteins, and therefore, purified F and G proteins have long been considered to be vaccine candidates. Suspensions of both F and G proteins have been prepared as purified proteins from various biological systems using mammalian cells, insect cells, and bacteria. Whole purified F and G protein preparations have been isolated from RSV-infected mammalian cell cultures using immunoaffinity or other chromatographic means. These purified proteins have been evaluated extensively in preclinical models and clinical trials. Rodent studies suggest that these subunit vaccines may induce an altered T-cell response, similar to that induced by FI-RSV, when used as the primary immunogenic in RSV-naive subjects.[57] In addition, these products are not thought to be immunogenic in young infants. Therefore, purified proteins are not likely to be good candidates for immunization of very young infants. They are well tolerated and moderately immunogenic at a 50-μg dose in older children and adults. These vaccines may be suitable for immunizing previously infected patients who are at high risk of severe disease during reinfection, such as children with bronchopulmonary dysplasia or cystic fibrosis, or the elderly.[26,45,58] These vaccines have also been considered for use in older children with asthma. In addition, such vaccines may prove to be useful in maternal immunization strategies.

A second subunit strategy under study has been the expression of F or G glycoproteins, or a novel FG chimeric molecule, from recombinant baculoviruses infecting insect cells. RSV antigens purified from these systems bind antibodies in human convalescent serum. The FG chimeric protein has been shown to induce a protective response in rodents. However, some safety concerns were raised when the FG chimera administered to rodents was associated with enhanced histopathology in some studies.[59]

A third strategy recently developed for subunit immunization is the expression of a portion of the G glycoprotein in a prokaryotic system (bacteria). The BB2GNa recombinant-derived protein contains a conserved polypeptide from RSV G protein fused to a streptococcal albumin-binding protein.[47] This subunit vaccine is immunogenic and protective in rodent studies, and phase I adult safety studies have been initiated.

Plasmid DNA vaccines. Virus proteins can be expressed in mammals following injection of plasmid cDNAs encoding virus genes into animals, particularly via the intramuscular route. Expression of reporter genes in muscle has been detected for months following administration in some cases. This approach might offer the advantage that protective antigens could be expressed in infants for a prolonged period, and might effectively immunize as maternal antibodies wane in the infant. Expression of the protein from cDNA within the cell, rather than administration of nonreplicating protein, also offers the potential advantage of loading class I MHC antigen presentation molecules with virus peptides for induction of CD8+ CTLs. Generally, the RSV F protein has not been well expressed from mammalian plasmid DNA vectors, but a recent report suggests that F encoded in newer expression vectors can induce a protective response in rodents.[48] The feasibility of this approach for use in humans remains to be determined.

Other approaches. Other novel approaches for vaccines to be used in infants, such as the use of peptides encoding antigenic epitopes and antigens incorporated in immune stimulating complex formulations (ISCOMS), have been investigated in limited laboratory and animal studies.[60] The Jennerian approach of using animal strains of RSV as vaccine candidates in humans has been proposed, but the protective antigens of these viruses are antigenically distinct from human RSV.[50] The use of novel adjuvants to augment or alter the type of immune response to RSV vaccine has also been investigated in animal models[61,62] and is under active investigation. Further investigation will be needed to evaluate the promise of all these approaches to RSV prevention.

Passive Immunization

Exogenously administered RSV-specific antibody. The successful clinical evaluation of both human polyclonal antibody and humanized murine monoclonal antibody has resulted in the licensure of human polyclonal intravenous immunoglobulin, RSV-IGIV (RespiGam™, MedImmune, Inc.), and the humanized monoclonal antibody, palivizumab (Synagis™, MedImmune, Inc.). These products validate earlier clinical observations suggesting that a serum-neutralizing antibody could protect against RSV disease.[20,63] These studies also demonstrated that high levels of serum-neutralizing antibody did not protect against RSV infection in the upper respiratory tract. The licensure of a humanized monoclonal antibody for widespread use in young infants represents a great step forward in the developing area of applied molecular biology and technology. Further refinements of this approach to passive immunization could be envisioned in the future, using novel modalities to permit more long-lasting or time-release of antibody to enable longer periods of antibody persistence without the expense and pain of multiple injections. Using inhaled antibody or antibody fragments to prevent RSV disease is also a possibility. Such products might also be evaluated for the treatment of RSV disease, although antiviral therapies have proven ineffective in the past, probably because virus shedding is already decreasing by the time a patient is hospitalized with RSV disease.

Maternal immunization. The availability of safe, purified RSV subunit vaccines, and the safety and efficacy of exogenously administered RSV polyclonal or monoclonal antibody have resulted in renewed interest in immunizing pregnant women to give full-term newborns high levels of RSV neutralizing antibodies.[14,64] Although the concept of immunizing a pregnant woman against RSV to help protect the infant raises significant safety concerns today, maternal immunization for other diseases has been used for decades. Maternal immunization is used to prevent both puerperal and neonatal tetanus in many countries throughout the world and immunization of pregnant women is recommended for several diseases, depending upon maternal health status and situation. For example, maternal immunization with live and inactivated polio vaccine has been well studied and may be recommended in a high-risk setting.[64,65] Trivalent inactivated influenza vaccine is also recommended for women who will be pregnant during the influenza season.[66]

Maternal immunization could be used to prevent serious disease in young infants who are at high risk for infections such as RSV and who are less responsive to most vaccines. In contrast to neonates, pregnant women respond well immunologically to most antigenic stimuli. Active maternal transfer of IgG antibody during the third trimester of pregnancy occurs physiologically. For example, cord concentrations of antibody directed against some antigens, such as tetanus, may actually exceed maternal antibody concentrations.[65] Vaccines administered late (the third trimester) in pregnancy are unlikely to be teratogenic or otherwise harmful to the fetus, but can result in the transfer of increased amounts of vaccine-specific antibody.[65] Importantly, pregnant women routinely seek medical care and are accessible for preventive interventions in both industrialized and developing countries. Since much of the cost involved in administering vaccines is related to patient accessibility, the cost of such a vaccination program would not be great. The cost of a theoretical maternal immunization program has been calculated to be significantly less than that for medical treatment of another, less common neonatal pathogen, group B *Streptococcus*.[66] Because the hospitalization rate for neonatal RSV disease is much higher than that for neonatal group B streptococcal infections (although the morbidity related to RSV is lower), an RSV maternal immunization program could be cost-effective if a safe, effective vaccine was available. The safety of maternally derived antibody would likely be greater than that of exogenously administered intravenous or intramuscular immunoglobulin, or even monoclonal antibody, at a greatly reduced cost. Importantly, immunizing a pregnant woman with a single dose of vaccine can potentially protect both the mother and baby by preventing or ameliorating maternal disease while conferring increased protection to the infant.[28] Maternal immunization may prevent maternal infection, thereby interrupting the chain of transmission to the baby, as well as directly protecting the baby by providing high levels of antibodies beginning at birth.

Another approach to augmenting maternal antibodies is the immunization of women before pregnancy, particularly if a vaccine stimulated a long-lasting antibody response. The use of maternal immunization combined with a live-attenuated RSV vaccine for the infant could also be considered if a safe and immunogenic candidate vaccine is developed, particularly a vaccine that would not be affected by maternal antibody. The possibility of immunizing pregnant women at approximately 32 to 35 weeks' gestation to provide the neonate with immunity at birth and then beginning active immunization at a slightly later age, perhaps at 2 months, could then be considered.

The immune responses in maternal sera and breast milk following administration of an experimental subunit RSV vaccine immediately after delivery (during the immediate postpartum period) have been evaluated in healthy women using the PFP-2 vaccine containing purified F fusion protein derived from the A2 strain of RSV (Wyeth-Lederle Pediatrics and Vaccines). A pilot study demonstrated that the PFP-2 vaccine was safe and immunogenic in postpartum women, resulting in high levels of RSV-specific antibody in the women and in their breast milk for at least 12 weeks following immunization.[28] A small, placebo-controlled, double-blind study of the PFP-2 vaccine in pregnant women is under way at the Baylor College of Medicine.

Maternal immunization against RSV is unlikely to be the sole solution for RSV prevention in infants. High-risk premature infants, particularly those born before 28 weeks' gestation, would be unlikely to benefit from maternal immunization because minimal maternal antibody (particularly little RSV-specific antibody) is transferred before that time.[28] Another potential adverse outcome could be immune inhibition of the subsequent response following active RSV immunization or disease. Activation or priming of the infant's immune system could occur, perhaps caused by the development of anti-idiotypic antibody to the maternal antibody. However, previous studies of other maternal vaccines have not demonstrated activation or priming of the infant's immune system following maternal immunization with influenza virus vaccine, tetanus toxoid vaccine, and *H influenzae* type b polysaccharide vaccine.[65,67]

Many of the concerns facing investigators interested in developing maternal vaccination are related to political and economic considerations. Many coincidental events occurring at birth or during the first months of life could be viewed as 'causal' or 'associated' by parents, clinicians, and lawyers. Factors such as the public's demand for 'no risk' medical care and the prevailing litigious climate, particularly in obstetrical and neonatal care, play a role in the reluctance of pharmaceutical companies to actively explore this avenue.[68]

Summary

RSV vaccines are not currently available for use in the general population or young children. New vaccine strategies need to be considered, and realistic goals must be set. Advances in molecular technology, vaccine adjuvants, and our understanding of immunologic mechanisms make the prospect of the prevention of RSV disease possible. While preventing all RSV infections may be neither realistic nor desirable, prevention of severe lower respiratory tract disease in young infants is a more reasonable, practical, and, perhaps, attainable goal. Any RSV vaccine strategy needs to use a vaccine that is relatively simple to administer, relatively inexpensive or easy to manufacture, and widely applicable to many populations. The most promising vaccine candidates include live-attenuated virus vaccines, and purified protein antigen vaccines. Live-attenuated virus vaccines, both biologically derived and genetically engineered, are good candidates for careful, sequential study in adults, children, and infants. If successful, these vaccines can be tested in other high-risk populations, such as premature infants, the elderly, or adults with chronic lung disease. Maternal immunization, perhaps using an RSV subunit vaccine, is an attractive model for examining the use of passive immunization in full-term infants. The possibility of immunizing pregnant women at approximately 35 weeks' gestation to provide the neonate with immunity at birth, followed by active immunization beginning at 2 months, is being considered. Approaches to the prevention of RSV disease in different patient populations may ultimately require both the use of various vaccines and prevention strategies to protect all individuals at high risk for sequelae of RSV infection.

References

1.   Prince GA, Horswood RL, Berndt J, et al: Respiratory syncytial virus infection in inbred mice. *Infect Immun* 1979;26:764-766.

2.   Graham BS, Perkins MD, Wright PF, et al: Primary respiratory syncytial virus infection in mice. *J Med Virol* 1988;26:153-162.

3.   Prince GA, Jenson AB, Horswood RL, et al: The pathogenesis of respiratory syncytial virus infection in cotton rats. *Am J Pathol* 1978;93:771-779.

4. Karron RA, Wright PF, Crowe JE Jr, et al: Evaluation of two live, cold-passaged, temperature-sensitive respiratory syncytial virus vaccines in chimpanzees and in human adults, infants, and children. *J Infect Dis* 1997;176:1428-1436.

5. Crowe JE Jr, Bui PT, Firestone CY, et al: Live subgroup B respiratory syncytial virus vaccines that are attenuated, genetically stable, and immunogenic in rodents and nonhuman primates. *J Infect Dis* 1996;173:829-839.

6. Wright PF, Karron RA, Belshe RB, et al: Evaluation of a live cold-passaged temperature-sensitive, respiratory syncytial virus (RSV) vaccine in infancy. *J Infect Dis* 2000. In press.

7. Anderson LJ, Hierholzer JC, Tsou C, et al: Antigenic characterization of respiratory syncytial virus strains with monoclonal antibodies. *J Infect Dis* 1985;151:626-633.

8. Johnson PR, Spriggs MK, Olmsted RA, et al: The G glycoprotein of human respiratory syncytial viruses of subgroups A and B: extensive sequence divergence between antigenically related proteins. *Proc Natl Acad Sci USA* 1987;84:5625-5629.

9. Belshe RB, Mendelman PM, Treanor J, et al: The efficacy of live-attenuated, cold-adapted, trivalent, intranasal influenza virus vaccine in children. *N Engl J Med* 1998;338:1405-1412.

10. Glezen WP, Paredes A, Allison JE, et al: Risk of respiratory syncytial virus infection for infants from low-income families in relationship to age, sex, ethnic group, and maternal antibody level. *J Pediatr* 1981;98:708-715.

11. McIntosh K, Halonen P, Ruuskanen O: Report of a workshop on respiratory viral infections: epidemiology, diagnosis, treatment, and prevention. *Clin Infect Dis* 1993;16:151-164.

12. Hall CB, Kopelman AE, Douglas RG, et al: Neonatal respiratory syncytial virus infection. *N Engl J Med* 1979;300:393-396.

13. Falsey AR, Treanor JJ, Betts RF, et al: Viral respiratory infections in the institutionalized elderly: clinical and epidemiologic findings. *J Am Geriatr Soc* 1992;140;115-119.

14. Englund JA: Passive protection against respiratory syncytial virus disease in infants: the role of maternal antibody. *Pediatr Infect Dis J* 1994;13:449-453.

15. Buraphacheep W, Sullender WM: The guinea pig as a model for the study of maternal immunization against respiratory syncytial virus infections in infancy. *J Infect Dis* 1997;175:935-938.

16. Crowe JE Jr, Bui PT, Siber GR, et al: Cold-passaged, temperature-sensitive mutants of human respiratory syncytial virus (RSV) are highly attenuated, immunogenic, and protective in seronegative chimpanzees, even when RSV antibodies are infused shortly before immunization. *Vaccine* 1995;13:847-855.

17. Reduction of respiratory syncytial virus hospitalization among premature infants and infants with bronchopulmonary dysplasia using respiratory syncytial virus immune globulin prophylaxis. The PREVENT Study Group. *Pediatrics* 1997;99:93-99.

18. Palivizumab, a humanized respiratory syncytial virus monoclonal antibody, reduces hospitalization from respiratory syncytial virus infection in high-risk infants.The IMpact-RSV Study Group. *Pediatrics* 1998;102:531-537.

19. Hall CB, Walsh EE, Long CE, et al: Immunity to and frequency of reinfection with respiratory syncytial virus. *J Infect Dis* 1991;163:693-698.

20. Glezen WP, Taber LH, Frank AL, et al: Risk of primary infection and reinfection with respiratory syncytial virus. *Am J Dis Child* 1986;140:543-546.

21. Kasel JA, Walsh EE, Frank AL, et al: Relation of serum antibody to glycoproteins of respiratory syncytial virus with immunity to infection in children. *Viral Immunol* 1987;1:199-205.

22. Kim HW, Canchola JG, Brandt CD, et al: Respiratory syncytial virus disease in infants despite poor administration of antigenic inactivated vaccine. *Am J Epidemiol* 1969;89:422-434.

23. Kapikian AZ, Mitchell RH, Chanock RM, et al: An epidemiologic study of altered clinical reactivity to respiratory syncytial (RS) virus infection in children previously vaccinated with an inactivated RS virus vaccine. *Am J Epidemiol* 1969;89:405-421.

24. Graham BS: Pathogenesis of respiratory syncytial virus vaccine-augmented pathology. *Am J Respir Crit Care Med* 1995;152:S63-S66.

25. Piedra PA, Grace S, Jewell A, et al: Sequential annual administration of purified fusion protein vaccine against respiratory syncytial virus in children with cystic fibrosis. *Pediatr Infect Dis J* 1998;17:217-224.

26. Groothuis JR, King SJ, Hogerman DA, et al: Safety and immunogenicity of a purified F protein respiratory syncytial virus

(PFP-2) vaccine in seropositive children with bronchopulmonary dysplasia. *J Infect Dis* 1998;177:467-469.

27. Falsey AR, Walsh EE: Safety and immunogenicity of a respiratory syncytial virus subunit vaccine (PFP-2) in ambulatory adults over age 60. *Vaccine* 1996;14:1214-1218.

28. Englund JA, Glezen WP, Piedra PA: Maternal immunization against viral disease. *Vaccine* 1998;16:1456-1463.

29. Cannon MJ, Openshaw PJ, Askonas BA: Cytotoxic T cells clear virus but augment lung pathology in mice infected with respiratory syncytial virus. *J Exp Med* 1988;168:1163-1168.

30. Wright PF, Shinozoki T, Fleet W, et al: Evaluation of a live, attenuated recombinant respiratory syncytial virus vaccine in infants. *J Pediatr* 1976;88:931-936.

31. King JC Jr, Burke AR, Clemens JD, et al: Respiratory syncytial virus illnesses in human immunodeficiency virus- and noninfected children. *Pediatr Infect Dis J* 1993;12:733-739.

32. Graham BS, Bunton LA, Wright PF, et al: Role of T lymphocyte subsets in the pathogenesis of primary infection and rechallenge with respiratory syncytial virus in mice. *J Clin Invest* 1991;88:1026-1033.

33. Muelanaer PM, Henderson FW, Hemming VG, et al: Group-specific serum antibody responses in children with primary and recurrent respiratory syncytial virus infections. *J Infect Dis* 1991;164:15-21.

34. Groothius JR, Simoes EAF, Levin MJ, et al: Prophylactic administration of respiratory syncytial virus immune globulin to high-risk infants and young children. *N Engl J Med* 1993;329:1524-1530.

35. McIntosh K, Masters HB, Orr I, et al: The immunologic response to infection with respiratory syncytial virus in infants. *J Infect Dis* 1978;138:24-32.

36. Mills J 5th, Van Kirk JE, Wright PF, et al: Experimental respiratory syncytial virus infection in adults. Possible mechanisms of resistance to infection and illness. *J Immunol* 1971;107:123-130.

37. Piedra PA, Glezen WP, Kasel JA, et al: Safety and immunogenicity of the PFP vaccine against respiratory syncytial virus (RSV): the western blot assay aids in distinguishing immune responses of the PFP vaccine from RSV infection. *Vaccine* 1995;13:1095-1101.

38. Murphy BR, Prince GA, Walsh EE, et al: Dissociation between serum neutralizing and glycoprotein antibody responses of infants and children who received inactivated respiratory syncytial virus vaccine. *J Clin Microbiol* 1986;24:197-202.

39. Crowe JE Jr: Current approaches to the development of vaccines against disease caused by respiratory syncytial virus (RSV) and parainfluenza virus (PIV). *Vaccine* 1995;13:415-421.

40. Dudas RA, Karron RA: Respiratory syncytial virus vaccines. *Clin Microbiol Rev* 1998;11:430-439.

41. Karron RA, Ambrosino DM: Respiratory syncytial virus vaccines. *Pediatr Infect Dis J* 1998;17:919-920.

42. Collins PL, Purcell RH, London WT, et al: Evaluation in chimpanzees of vaccinia virus recombinants that express the surface glycoproteins of human respiratory syncytial virus. *Vaccine* 1990;8:164-168.

43. Wyatt LS, Whitehead SS, Venanzi KA, et al: Priming and boosting immunity to respiratory syncytial virus by recombinant replication defective vaccinia virus MVA. *Vaccine* 1999;18:392-397.

44. Hsu KH, Lubeck MD, Davis AR, et al: Immunogenicity of recombinant adenovirus-RSV vaccines with adenovirus types 4, 5, and 7 vectors in dogs and a chimpanzee. *J Infect Dis* 1992;166:769-775.

45. Piedra PA, Grace S, Jewell A, et al: Purified fusion protein vaccine protects against lower respiratory tract illness during respiratory syncytial virus season in children with cystic fibrosis. *Pediatr Infect Dis J* 1996;15:23-31.

46. Wathen MW, Brideau RJ, Thomsen DR: Immunization of cotton rats with the human respiratory syncytial virus F glycoprotein produced using a baculovirus vector. *J Infect Dis* 1989;159:255-264.

47. Power UF, Plotnicky-Gilquin H, Huss T, et al: Induction of protective immunity in rodents by vaccination with a prokaryotically expressed recombinant fusion protein containing a respiratory syncytial virus G protein fragment. *Virology* 1997;230:155-166.

48. Li X, Sambhara S, Li CX, et al: Protection against respiratory syncytial virus infection by DNA immunization. *J Exp Med* 1998;188:681-688.

49. Chargelegue D, Obeid OE, Hse SC, et al: A peptide mimic of a protective epitope of respiratory syncytial virus selected from a combinatorial library induces virus-neutralizing antibodies and reduces viral load in vivo. *J Virol* 1998;72:2040-2046.

50. Piazza FM, Johnson SA, Darnell ME, et al: Bovine respiratory syncytial virus protects cotton rats against human respiratory syncytial virus infection. *J Virol* 1993;67:1503-1510.

51. Karron RA, Wright PF, Newman FK, et al: A live human parainfluenza type 3 virus vaccine is attenuated and immunogenic in healthy infants and children. *J Infect Dis* 1995;172:1445-1450.

52. Collins PL, Hill MG, Camargo E, et al: Production of infectious human respiratory syncytial virus from cloned cDNA confirms an essential role for the transcription elongation factor from the 5' proximal open reading frame of the M2 mRNA in gene expression and provides a capability for vaccine development. *Proc Natl Acad Sci USA* 1995;92:11563-11567.

53. Crowe JE Jr, Firestone CY, Collins PL, et al: Acquisition of the ts phenotype by a chemically mutagenized cold-passaged human respiratory syncytial virus vaccine candidate results from the acquisition of a single mutation in the polymerase (L) gene. *Virus Genes* 1996;13:269-273.

54. Firestone CY, Whitehead S, Collins PL, et al: Nucleotide sequence analysis of the respiratory syncytial virus (RSV) subgroup A cold-passaged (cp), temperature sensitive (ts) cpts-248/404 live-attenuated virus vaccine candidate. *Virology* 1996;225:419-422.

55. Collins PL, Whitehead SS, Bukreyev A, et al: Rational design of live-attenuated recombinant vaccine virus for human respiratory syncytial virus by reverse genetics. *Adv Virus Res* 1999;54:423-451.

56. Crowe JE Jr, Collins PL, London WT, et al: A comparison in chimpanzees of the immunogenicity and efficacy of live-attenuated respiratory syncytial virus (RSV) temperature-sensitive mutant vaccines and vaccinia virus recombinants that express the surface glycoproteins of RSV. *Vaccine* 1993;11:1395-1404.

57. Murphy BR, Sotnikov AV, Lawrence LA, et al: Enhanced pulmonary histopathology is observed in cotton rats immunized with formalin-inactivated respiratory syncytial virus (RSV) or purified F glycoprotein and challenged with RSV 3-6 months after immunization. *Vaccine* 1990;8:497-502.

58. Falsey AR, Walsh EE: Safety and immunogenicity of a respiratory syncytial virus subunit vaccine (PFP-2) in the institutionalized elderly. *Vaccine* 1997;15:1130-1132.

59. Connors M, Collins PL, Firestone CY, et al: Cotton rats previously immunized with a chimeric RSV FG glycoprotein develop enhanced pulmonary pathology when infected with RSV, a phenomenon not encountered following immunization with vaccinia-RSV recombinants or RSV. *Vaccine* 1992;10:475-484.

60. Hu KF, Elvander M, Merza M, et al: The immunostimulating complex (ISCOM) is an efficient mucosal delivery system for respiratory syncytial virus (RSV) envelope antigens inducing high local and systemic antibody responses. *Clin Exp Immunol* 1998;113:235-243.

61. Hancock GE, Speelman DJ, Frenchick PJ, et al: Formulation of the purified fusion protein of respiratory syncytial virus with the saponin QS-21 induces protective immune responses in Balb/c mice that are similar to those generated by experimental infection. *Vaccine* 1995;13:391-400.

62. Neuzil KM, Johnson JE, Tang YW, et al: Adjuvants influence the quantitative and qualitative immune response in BALB/c mice immunized with respiratory syncytial virus FG subunit vaccine. *Vaccine* 1997;15:525-532.

63. Walsh EE, Schlesinger JJ, Brandriss MW: Protection from respiratory syncytial virus infection in cotton rats by passive transfer of monoclonal antibodies. *Infect Immun* 1984;43:756-758.

64. Englund JA, Glezen WP: Maternal immunization for the prevention of infection in early infancy. *Semin Pediatr Infect Dis* 1991;2:225-231.

65. Englund JA, Mbawuike IN, Hammill H, et al: Maternal immunization with influenza or tetanus toxoid vaccine for passive antibody protection in young infants. *J Infect Dis* 1993;168:647-656.

66. CDC: Advisory Committee on Immunization Practices. Prevention and control of influenza. *MMWR Morb Mortal Wkly Rep* 1998;47:1-26.

67. Glezen WP, Englund JA, Siber GR, et al: Maternal immunization with the capsular polysaccharide vaccine for *H influenzae* type b. *J Infect Dis* 1992;165(suppl):S134-S136.

68. Baker CJ: Immunization to prevent group B streptococcal disease: Victories and vexation. *J Infect Dis* 1990;161:917-921.

Chapter **11**

The Economics of RSV Infection, Prevention, and Treatment

Albert Marchetti, MD

Medical Director and Vice President
Health Economics Research,
Division of Physicians World Communications Group

Eric A. F. Simoes, MD, DCH

Affiliated with University of Colorado
Health Sciences Center
Associate Professor, Pediatrics,
Department of Pediatric Infectious Diseases

Respiratory syncytial virus (RSV) is the most common pathogen of the respiratory tract and the most important etiologic agent of lower respiratory tract infections in neonates, infants, and young children.[1-3] During the first year of life, 40% to 80% of the pediatric population of the United States may become infected,[2-4] approximately 1% of infected infants (100,000 babies per year) will require hospital care for severe disease, and about 2% of these (2,000 babies per year) will die from the infection and related complications.[3,5] Worldwide, the incidence of RSV infection is proportionally greater, with more than 500,000 RSV-related deaths occurring annually at untold cost.[6]

Several factors—including smoking in the home, crowding in the home, daycare, and lower socioeconomic background—predispose children to increased risk for RSV infection.[1,7] Constitutional factors—including prematurity, postpartum chronologic age <6 months, chronic lung disease, congenital heart disease, cystic fibrosis, and immunodeficiencies—predispose children to more severe RSV infection, a higher rate of associated complications, and increased mortality.[8-13] For mild self-limiting infections, supportive home care is the mainstay of therapy. For moderate-to-severe infections and for distinct subsets of patients, hospitalization with extensive resource utilization is often required.

Disease prevention to avert the morbidity and mortality caused by RSV infection and to reduce the associated economic burden is preferable to treatment. No RSV vaccine to protect neonates and infants has been successfully developed to date.[14-20] Prophylactic, intravenous RSV immune globulin (RSV-IGIV, RespiGam™) is safe and effective, and has been shown to reduce RSV-related hospitalizations in high-risk infants since its introduction into clinical practice.[21,22] Likewise, the safety and efficacy of a monoclonal antibody against RSV (palivizumab, Synagis™) were established in clinical trials with at-risk pediatric populations.[23] Intramuscular palivizumab has generally replaced intravenous RSV-IGIV for routine clinical care, except, possibly, among children with severe bronchopulmonary dysplasia or deficiencies that require treatment with immunoglobulin.[24]

Because intravenous RSV-IGIV and intramuscular palivizumab are costly and the population of infants at risk is large, concern about the affordability of RSV prophylaxis has been expressed by some health-care providers and payers. However, concern over the cost of RSV treatment for infected infants and children, especially those hospitalized with severe illness, is also occasionally raised when health-care system budgets and operational expenses are reviewed. Moreover, the use of the antiviral ribavirin (Virazole®), bronchodilators, and corticosteroids has been questioned because of cost and lack of positive evidence regarding their effectiveness. Such questions necessitate health economic research to determine the clinical and economic impact of RSV infection, as well as the costs and consequences of currently available prophylactic, diagnostic, and therapeutic interventions. Unfortunately, the general lack of familiarity with the methodologies of health economics hampers widespread understanding of the costs and benefits of resources dedicated to disease management. To date, published research has revealed: 1) limitations in availability and reliability of RSV-related data; 2) complexity and variability of infection and individual patient care; and 3) diversity of hospitalization rates and costs associated with disease management. Each of these topics will be explored in this chapter, starting with an overview of some basic concepts in health economics.

Value in Health Care

In the 20th century, as diagnostic, therapeutic, and prophylactic interventions became increasingly sophisticated and widely available, the quality of health care became synonymous with the quantity or intensity of care dedicated to individual patients. Treatments were delivered under the assumption that they were scientifically justified and clinically relevant, and health-care value was thought to be inherent in all services, principally as a function of safety and efficacy. However, with early health insurance cost-containment programs came skepticism over the appropriateness of some therapeutic interventions, particularly surgical procedures. Insurers developed lists of potentially overused interventions and commissioned studies into the frequency of unnecessary treatments. The growth of utilization reviews and second-opinion programs promoted the idea that not all treatments were effectively or appropriately used. Moreover, studies showed considerable geographic variation in clinical practice, predominantly based on differences in professional training, physician skills, and local or regional practice patterns, rather than patient variability.

As the concept that health-care value is implicit in all treatment programs was slowly dispelled, evidence of quality and value in health care was demanded. Clinical evaluations were instituted to demonstrate real-world effectiveness, and economic evaluations were required to demonstrate cost justification. The melding of clinical and economic methodologies yielded a new discipline, health economics, which has since served to explicate the value of health-care products and practices, both old and new, and to promote the optimal use of available resources.

To optimize clinical practice, care must be efficient and without ethical compromise. In other words, providers must deliver the most effective services that produce the greatest impact at the smallest cost, and on such a scale that incremental expenses are justified by incremental benefits.[25] These concepts are at the core of health economics, and convey the essential principles of value.

Defining the quality of a treatment as its effectiveness or utility, and assigning a cost to achieve that quality (assessing cost-effectiveness, for example) is the same as determining value. Current health economic research attempts to evaluate interventions and technologies for cost-effectiveness, cost-benefit, and appropriateness under real-world conditions. Manufacturers commonly commission health economic studies in conjunction with clinical trials to demonstrate the economic value, safety, and efficacy of their products. Studies conducted by individual payers and providers help to illuminate costs and benefits in defined health-care environments (eg, hospitals, departments, managed care plans), and can reveal the potential for profit and loss based on the levels of resource utilization and reimbursement.

Perspective

A health economic study can be conducted from a single perspective (point of view) or from multiple perspectives. Common points of view include those of the patient, provider, payer, and society. Although the outcomes to be evaluated are generally consistent across perspectives, the costs are not.

Patients: Costs from the patient's perspective include those portions of the total charges for care that are not covered by insurance (ie, deductibles, copayments, and nonreimbursable expenses). For patients without insurance, costs are equivalent to the full charges for those products and services that are received during the course of an illness. In addition to medically related costs, patients also bear indirect and intangible costs that are incurred throughout the illness. Lost work productivity and lost wages, as well as expenses incurred in accessing care and the monetary value of pain and suffering also contribute to the total cost of care from the patient's perspective. Consequences from the patient's perspective are the clinical effects or outcomes and adverse events experienced with or without medical or surgical intervention.

Providers: Providers can be hospitals, clinics, home health-care agencies, long-term care facilities, managed-care organizations, and individual and group practices. Costs from the provider's perspective are the expenses incurred during the provision of care. These costs may include expenditures for drugs, laboratory tests, equipment, supplies, insurance, maintenance, and the physical facility where care is given, as well as the salaries of health-care workers and office staff. These are the provider's contributions to the products and services supplied to patients. Information on the actual cost of a service may be difficult to obtain. Charge data may be more readily available, but are often not reflective of the true costs from the provider's perspective. Profit or loss is equal to reimbursement minus the cost.

Payers: The cost to payers (insurers) is defined as reimbursable charges for products and services delivered to patients. As with providers, primary costs from the payer's perspective are direct, not indirect or intangible. Payers may reimburse providers or patients in part or in full, depending on previously arranged contracts and policies, or pre-established standards within the industry.

Society: Costs from the societal perspective include patient morbidity and mortality costs, and the full expense of giving and receiving medical care. Included are direct medical and nonmedical expenses, as well as indirect expenses (eg, lost productivity or wages) and intangible costs (eg, pain and suffering).

Types of Health Economic Analyses

The fundamental objectives of health economic evaluation are to identify, measure, and compare the costs and consequences of alternative management options for patient care. The common types of studies are: cost of illness, cost minimization, cost-benefit, cost-effectiveness, and cost-utility analyses.

Cost of illness/burden of disease: In cost-of-illness evaluations, the overall costs (direct and indirect) associated with a specific disease or illness are determined. Quite often, painstaking analyses of epidemiologic data are required, along with reviews of claims databases or institutional medical charts that span the continuum of care for patients with a particular condition. The results are expressed in dollars. The baseline cost data generated by these studies can be used to estimate the economic value of treatment, for example, the dollar benefit of a treatment that alters the natural history of an illness.

Cost minimization: Cost minimization is used to compare 2 or more health-care alternatives that are equal in effectiveness (ie, they produce similar clinical outcomes). This type of analysis compares the cost of competing interventions. Outcomes need not be evaluated because of the underlying assumption of clinical equivalence. The results are expressed in dollars.

Cost-benefit: In a cost-benefit analysis, the monetary benefits realized from a product or service are compared with the costs of providing that product or service. The results are typically expressed as a cost-benefit ratio, a net cost, or a net benefit. If the clinical outcomes related to an intervention can be measured in dollars, a cost-benefit analysis can be performed. This type of analysis is commonly used to evaluate illness prevention programs.

Cost-effectiveness: A cost-effectiveness analysis is useful when comparing treatment alternatives or competing management options that differ in cost and achieved clinical outcomes. In such analyses, costs are measured in dollars, while outcomes are measured and expressed in natural units, such as millimeter reductions in blood pressure, disease-free days, clinical success (intermediate outcomes), and mortality or quality of life (terminal outcomes). These analyses seek to identify alternatives that yield the best health-care outcome per dollar spent. Results are expressed as a cost-effectiveness ratio for each comparator.

Cost-utility: Cost-utility is an economic concept that relates to the subjective value of an outcome, unlike the objective clinical value that is used in a cost-effectiveness study or the dollar value that is used in a cost-benefit study. In cost-utility analyses, the cost of a treatment is expressed in dollars, while the outcome or clinical consequence is expressed in terms of patient preference, satisfaction, willingness to pay, quality-adjusted life years, or other somewhat subjective measures. This type of assessment is useful when evaluating alternative interventions that extend life or reduce morbidity. The results of cost-utility analyses are often expressed as cost per quality-adjusted life year gained.

Decision Analysis

A decision analysis is frequently used to structure the logical and chronological order of medical decisions, as well as related resource utilization and outcomes achievement. Decision analyses are systematic quantitative methods of describing clinical problems, identifying potential courses of action, assessing the probability and value of likely outcomes, and making a calculation to identify the optimum course of action.

A tool frequently used in decision analysis is a decision tree or simulation model that enables investigators to graphically display all interventional alternatives being compared, the outcomes associated with each, and the probability of their occurrence within specific patient populations (Figure 1). The tree provides the basis for an algebraic conversion of all variables into one summary measurement, for example, a cost-effectiveness or cost-benefit ratio that allows 2 or more health-care alternatives to be compared.

Conducting Health Economic Research

The design and conduct of health economic research generally require a combination of methodologies that are implemented in a sequential fashion. Initially, a research question is posed in an answerable form from a specific perspective. Next, a clinical assessment is performed to identify the components of care that are dedicated to individual patients and the anticipated outcomes with patient management. Subsequently, a model is created to schematically represent the clinical pathways through which patients progress in order to achieve the desired outcomes. Resource utilization and costs are then identified for each pathway. Finally, analyses are performed to answer the research question and to determine the strength of results (sensitivity calculations). Although not all steps are required for all studies, the basic principles and methods are maintained and applied as needed.

RSV Infection and Patient Management

Research perspectives and questions related to RSV infection and patient management are as diverse as the

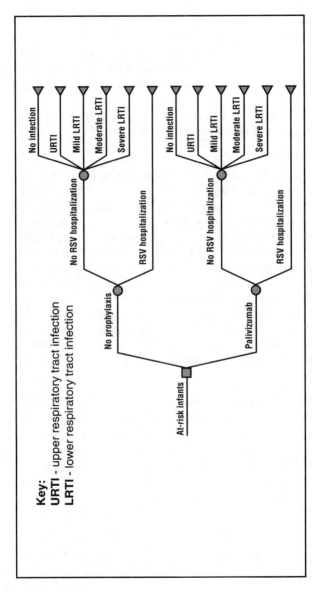

Key:
URTI - upper respiratory tract infection
LRTI - lower respiratory tract infection

No infection
URTI
Mild LRTI
Moderate LRTI
Severe LRTI

No RSV hospitalization
RSV hospitalization

No infection
URTI
Mild LRTI
Moderate LRTI
Severe LRTI

No RSV hospitalization
RSV hospitalization

No prophylaxis
Palivizumab

At-risk infants

Figure 1: Decision analysis model (Decision tree)

clinical practices that are used to protect, diagnose, and treat at-risk children. Individual patient factors, and the severity and complexity of their infections, as well as provider preferences and regional practice patterns, all influence clinical management decisions and related resource utilization. Consequently, health economic research into RSV disease management must comprehensively and credibly account for such variations.

Diagnosis

During the RSV season, infants and children with respiratory tract symptoms are probably infected with RSV.[26-29] At other times of the year, other etiologies are more probable.[27,28] Identifying the etiologic agent is academic in most cases (except for hospital cohorting to prevent nosocomial RSV spread), because the common signs and symptoms of infection will direct individual patient care, which is generally supportive and not specific to RSV.[1] However, when a diagnosis is required, it can be made with near certainty by testing nasopharyngeal aspirates or washes for RSV antigens (immunofluorescence or enzyme-linked immunosorbent assays), by qualitatively searching for genetic material (PCR), or by growing live virions (viral culture).[3,24,30]

Patient Management

Mild-to-moderate RSV infections are generally self-limiting, but can be complicated by acute otitis media and secondary bacterial infection. Supportive home care with or without minimal professional intervention is sufficient management for most patients. Recovery from the acute episode is expected within 3 to 7 days.

RSV infection may lead to more serious lower respiratory tract illnesses (ie, croup, bronchiolitis, and pneumonia) that require closer attention and greater resource utilization. Signs of LRT involvement, such as coughing, wheezing, and breathing with difficulty and/or retractions, usually follow upper respiratory tract infections in a few days. Bronchiolitis and associated acute respiratory distress may worsen. Inhaled bronchodilators (eg, salbutamol, epinephrine) may lead to limited clinical improvement for a minority of patients by relieving bronchospasm, respiratory distress, and related hypoxia, but probably will not reduce the frequency of hospitalizations.[31-33] For this reason, inhaled bronchodilators are infrequently used in outpatient clinical practices; economic analyses of these practices have not been conducted.

Ribavirin Therapy

For hospitalized infants with RSV-related bronchiolitis, ribavirin therapy (the only FDA-approved antiviral therapy for RSV) provides little or no clinical benefit, and does not definitively reduce length of hospital stay for infected patients.[34,35] Some evidence of effectiveness in hospitalized infants on oxygen and ventilation has been demonstrated.[36] However, conflicting evidence comes from other studies that note similar or incremental resource utilization.[37-42] Possible causes for the conflicting results include heterogeneous research groups, small patient numbers in some studies, and varied criteria for clinical outcomes. Regardless, these studies have raised probing questions about the use of ribavirin in children with serious RSV infections and, consequently, have significantly limited its use. Moreover, because overall health-care expenditures related to ribavirin use have not been fully elucidated, cost-benefit has not been established. Economic considerations are discussed elsewhere in this chapter.

Steroid Therapy

Steroids have not been definitively shown to alter the acute clinical course or long-term sequelae related to RSV infection.[43-45] Acute outcomes of interest—duration of hospital stay, drug utilization, and supportive care—were not diminished with steroid use, nor were the first-year follow-up outcomes of morbidity, drug utilization, and frequency of positive allergy testing in a placebo-controlled study with 147 infants.[44] In another study involving infants 2 years of age hospitalized with acute bronchiolitis, 65 who received dexamethasone did not experience reduced oxygen therapy or reduced time to resolution of symptoms, compared with 53 who did not receive the steroid.[45] Likewise, in a smaller (N=29) double-blind, placebo-controlled dexamethasone efficacy study, no immediately significant differences in respiratory rate, oxygen saturation, clinical score, or pulmonary function were noted between groups.[43] Based on currently available evidence, steroids should not be administered to infants or children with RSV lower respiratory tract infection.

Supportive Therapies

Inpatient care for RSV infection frequently encompasses close monitoring of the infant, adequate hydration, and oxygen administration to correct hypoxia. In more severe cases, infants may require mechanical ventilation. The percentage of infants hospitalized for RSV infection who require supplemental oxygen and mechanical ventilation has been reported in the literature at rates of 37% to 71%, and 0.2% to 38%, respectively, depending on such factors as age and associated comorbidities.[23,46,47]

Oxygen

Humidified oxygen is indicated for hospitalized infants who are hypoxic, dyspneic, or cyanotic. Hypoxia is present if oxygen saturation of arterial blood is <88% in neonates and <90% in infants older than 28 days; or if arterial oxygen tension is <50 torr in neonates and <60 torr in infants older than 28 days.[48] Oxygen may also help decrease insensible water loss from tachypnea.[49] Oxygenation should be closely monitored to avoid potential complications, such as retinopathy of prematurity in infants <35 weeks' gestation, ventilatory depression, oxygen toxicity, absorption atelectasis, and depression of ciliary and/or leukocytic function.[48]

Ventilation

For severely ill patients with significant apnea, severe oxygen desaturation, progressive or persistent acidosis, or respiratory insufficiency/failure, mechanical ventilation may need to be integrated into patient management. Patients may also require intubation, depending on the state of consciousness, arterial oxygen saturation, and partial arterial carbon dioxide pressure. As with initiation of supplemental oxygen therapy, mechanical ventilation should be closely monitored to ensure adequate lung inflation, and to avoid potential complications.[50] Prolonged ventilation should also be avoided when possible, since risks of comorbidity and ventilator dependency are potential adverse outcomes.[51] At a per unit charge of $1,152 per day,[52] mechanical ventilation is a costly component of RSV hospitalization.

Antibiotics

RSV infections are not treated with antibiotics, but antibiotics may be prescribed if evidence of otitis media or secondary bacterial infection is noted. Generally occurring in less than 2% of all RSV hospitalized infants,[53] secondary bacterial infections are evidenced by the clinical deterioration of the patient (with or without sepsis), atypical radiologic evidence, positive gram stains or culture, sensitivity tests on tracheal samples, and higher white blood cell counts with immature forms.[49] The cost of antibiotic therapy varies according to infant and the presence of comorbidities at the time of treatment.

Hospitalization

Most infants and young children with moderate-to-severe disease are best managed as inpatients, because RSV infection is occasionally associated with life-threatening complications that require intensive care. Hospitalization rates for RSV infection range from 1% to 45%, depending on patient characteristics and environmental factors.[2,11,21,54] Rates may also vary with the severity of annual epidemics. Prematurity, postpartum chronologic age <6 months, chronic lung disease, congenital heart disease, cystic fibrosis, and immunodeficiency predispose children to more severe RSV infection, a higher rate of associated complications, more frequent hospitalizations, and increased mortality.[8-13,46,55,56] The need for hospitalization can be generally assessed on the basis of: 1) responsiveness; 2) ability to feed; 3) hydration; and 4) oxygenation.[57] Moreover, if the quality of familial care is dubious or the nutrition of the child is questionable, hospitalization is the prudent choice.

Among hospitalized infants and children, bronchiolitis was the most common admitting diagnosis (37.4%) in a clinical profile of 246 pediatric patients who were hospitalized in a tertiary-care center in California.[58] Pneumonia (32.5%) and possible septicemia (13%) were other frequent admitting diagnoses. The median age of infected patients was 3 months; median length of stay was 3 days. Fifteen percent of patients required intensive care, and 76% required ventilation assistance. Patients with underlying cardiopulmonary disease had a longer duration of intensive care and prolonged hospital stays.

An international retrospective study by chart review conducted by Behrendt et al revealed that the median length of stay for infants with documented RSV infections was approximately 4 days in the United States, United Kingdom, Australia, and Finland.[59] In these countries, children may be discharged on oxygen and prescribed other forms of ancillary home care. In most European countries, with Finland as the only exception, hospitalizations lasted 8 to 9 days (median length of stay), since infants were discharged only after they had completely recovered. Regardless of length of hospital stay, patient management varied by country, as well as by care center, and appeared independent of patient characteristics and clinical status (Table 1).

RSV Prophylaxis

For children at high risk for severe RSV infection, hospitalization, and high resource consumption, intravenous RSV-specific immune globulin (RSV-IGIV, RespiGam™) and intramuscular monoclonal antibody (palivizumab, Synagis™) can be administered for protection.[21-23] In 2 multicenter trials with RSV-IGIV, prophylaxed infants with underlying illnesses, such as bronchopulmonary dysplasia or congenital heart disease, and those born prematurely or infected at a very early age (<6 months), incurred fewer RSV-related hospital admissions and bed and intensive care days when compared with unprophylaxed controls. They also contracted otitis media less frequently.[60] The American Academy of Pediatrics suggests that neonates who require oxygen for severe bronchopulmonary dysplasia and those with immune deficiencies may derive added benefit from RSV-IGIV prophylaxis because of its broader coverage against non-RSV respiratory tract infection. However, infants with cyanotic congenital heart disease should not be given RSV-IGIV, because they may experience serious adverse events associated with cardiac surgery.

Currently, for most clinical scenarios, palivizumab (Synagis™) is preferred over RSV-IGIV (RespiGam™) because of its greater convenience and ease of use. A randomized, double-blind, placebo-controlled study conducted during the 1996-1997 RSV season showed that palivizumab is safe and effective for the prevention of RSV-related hospitalization of at-risk infants.[23] A 55% reduction in the RSV-related hospitalization rate for the palivizumab group (4.8%) compared with the placebo group (10.6%) was documented, along with fewer over-

Table 1: Resource Utilization List for Consumables Related to Inpatient Care

Inpatient Care

- Hospital bed days
- Emergency department (ED)
- ED supplies
- NICU
- NICU nursing
- NICU supplies
- Isolated NICU
- PICU
- PICU nursing
- PICU supplies
- Isolated PICU
- ICU—nonspecialized
- ICU nursing
- ICU supplies
- Isolated ICU
- SCU
- SCU nursing
- SCU supplies
- Isolated SCU
- Ambulance
- Helicopter
- Ward
- Ward nursing
- Ward supplies
- Isolated ward

KEY:

NICU- neonatal intensive care unit
PICU- pediatric intensive care unit
SCU- special care unit

Physician Services
- Hospital ward attending physician
- ED physician
- ICU physician
- Resident
- SCU attending physician
- Neonatologist
- Speech/language specialist
- Hematologist
- Ophthalmologist
- Neonatal nurse practitioner (NNP)
- Social worker
- Case manager
- Lactation consultant
- Occupational therapist
- Respiratory therapist

Radiology
- Chest x-ray

Diagnostic Tests
Main Tests
- Enzyme immunoassay
- PCR
- Cell culture

Others:
- Urine culture
- CSF culture
- Blood culture
- Viral culture
- Antibody screen

Laboratory Tests
Main Tests
- Blood gas analysis
- Chem 7
- CBC count with differential
- Urinalysis
- Electrolytes

Others:
- Type and cross
- Nasal wash
- IgG
- Blood type RBC phenotype
- Hgb/HTC
- Glucose

all hospital days, fewer days of serious illness, and decreased oxygen requirements. Intensive care unit and mechanical ventilation days were similar between the groups. Adverse events were low and similar to those observed with placebo. In a prospective, international, single-arm, open-label trial, 565 patients were enrolled in 77 centers and received monthly injections of palivizumab throughout the RSV season.[61] The hospitalization rate of patients who were untested or had confirmed RSV disease was 3.7%. A subsequent retrospective outcomes assessment conducted by chart review (N=1839) in the United States indicated that 2.3% of patients who received palivizumab were hospitalized for confirmed RSV illness.[62]

Economics

For economic analyses of RSV prevention and related complications and/or sequelae of infection, a perspective must be selected before the study is designed and implemented. Objectives and time horizons must be established, and a research question should be posed. Direct medical expenditures can be assessed for all products and services that are consumed during inpatient and outpatient care. Direct nonmedical costs for travel, lodging, food, and other child care, as well as the indirect costs associated with losses (productivity and wages) that are incurred by parental or familial caregivers of infected children, can be included. Moreover, intangible costs related to the emotional impact of a sick child on other family members, although difficult to calculate, can at least be acknowledged in the total health economic equation. Each of these costs—direct, indirect, and intangible—contributes to the total economic burden of RSV infection on society, but may not be appropriate to include in every analysis because objectives and perspectives vary.

Previous studies have elucidated various aspects of the economics of RSV infection, and some general impressions have emerged. Areas of particular interest include the costs associated with ribavirin therapy; the costs and consequences of RSV-specific prophylaxis with RSV-IGIV and intramuscular palivizumab; and the frequency, intensity, duration, and cost of institutional and ambulatory care. Additionally, the potential link of early moderate-to-severe RSV infection and subsequent reactive airway disease has spurred economic interest because such a link would enhance the value of RSV prophylactic and treatment modalities. Each of these topics will be explored in the remainder of this chapter.

Ribavirin

In view of its cost and questionable effectiveness, ribavirin (Virazole®) is restricted to patients with severe disease who face sizable risk of mortality. The cost of aerosolized ribavirin is $480 per dose in the United States, which is substantial, but could be offset if potential reductions in the use of other resources, in ICU time, or in overall length of hospital stay could be proved. To date, such reductions have not been demonstrated conclusively; in fact, some studies documented increased resource consumption associated with ribavirin use. A small cost study (N=44) was performed using 2 matched cohorts of RSV-infected children.[39] Significantly longer ICU time and a significantly protracted hospital course with increased resource utilization were noted for the ribavirin group. Translated into immediate health-care expenditures, these differences amounted to an average per-patient cost of $15,552 for those in the ribavirin group, compared with $5,156 for those in the control group. However, extrapolation of these results to broader patient populations should be done with caution.

The projected incremental spending for ribavirin could be offset by downstream cost savings if long-term clinical benefits followed use of the drug in the early acute setting. Indeed, longer-term outcome studies were conducted, but have not consistently demonstrated clinical benefits related to ribavirin use among seriously ill hospitalized infants with RSV infection.[38,63-67] Therefore, economic analyses based on these studies would be inconsistent.

To confidently assess the economic impact of ribavirin on RSV disease management, data on institutional care, on resource consumption, and on length of hospital stay are essential, as is information on ribavirin's potential to reduce the frequency of chronic reactive airway disease later in life. Information on mortality is also important for economic evaluations and absolutely paramount for proving clinical and societal benefit. Comparative cost-in-use studies and cost-effectiveness analyses of ribavirin therapy remain to be conducted; however, the likelihood of such studies is minimal in light of insufficient clinical benefit.

RSV-Specific Prophylaxis

As previously discussed, the clinical benefit of immune prophylaxis against RSV infection has been well established.[22,23] Economic questions principally relate to the likelihood of incremental expenses or the potential for cost savings associated with such intervention. For example: is the cost of prophylaxing all infants at risk for RSV infection greater or less than the cost of treating RSV infections and subsequent sequelae for all infants who become infected? If incremental costs are incurred with prophylaxis, are they reasonable for the expected short- or long-term health benefits derived? To answer these questions, 2 important variables must be quantified: 1) the probability of RSV-related hospitalizations among at-risk children, and 2) the costs associated with hospital and ambulatory care of infected children. Independently and collectively, these variables strongly influence health economic assessments, and are the driving factors in the economics of RSV infection from the payer and provider perspectives. If the factors of direct nonmedical costs, indirect costs associated with infection, and the probability of developing chronic reactive airway disease after previous severe RSV infection are added, the framework is established for a complete economic assessment from the societal perspective.

Seasonal Probability of RSV Infection and Hospitalization Among Children at Risk

Incidence rates of RSV infection vary substantially among clinical studies and epidemiologic reports. They are affected by the extent of RSV diagnostic testing to establish an etiology for infections, regional/seasonal severity,[68-70] RSV strain and subspecies virulence,[71-73] institutional divergence in quality of neonatal care,[74-76] and various socioeconomic factors, such as crowding and cigarette smoking in the home.[7,77,78] Estimated hospitalization rates for respiratory infections among premature infants range from 41 admissions per 100 child years,[79] to 85 admissions per 100 child years.[10] As a causative agent, RSV accounts for 42% to 79% of all reported infections,[80-82] and 100% of infections evaluated in RSV clinical trials. (RSV studies in which a definitive diagnosis is not required may contain non-RSV patients.)[21-23]

A prospective 2-year study of respiratory rehospitalization rates for premature infants (<32 weeks' gestation) revealed a 36% rehospitalization rate for respiratory illnesses following initial hospital discharge.[11] For matched full-term infants, the rehospitalization rate was 2.5%. In a separate analysis of resources consumed by preterm infants after initial hospital discharge, an ancillary finding indicated that approximately 55% were readmitted with respiratory infections.[79] Estimates of RSV-related hospitalizations for nonprophylaxed preterm infants vary, with rates of 10.6%,[23] 13.5%,[22] 20.7%,[79] 22.4%,[21] 36%,[11] and 42.6% reported.[10] Some factors that may account for these differences include: the severity of the RSV season; viral subspecies; nature of the at-risk population; and urban vs rural location. In recent years, lower hospitalization rates were observed in some high-risk groups, which may reflect improved parental education and widespread use of RSV prophylaxis for targeted risk groups.

The Cost of RSV-Related Hospitalization

When all potential direct medical costs are viewed together, the hospitalization expenses are the largest, constituting about 62% of total direct medical costs, based on Canadian data.[83] Physician fees constitute about 4% of costs, and ambulatory care accounts for 38% of total direct medical expenditures in Canada. Thus, the greatest potential for direct medical cost savings in RSV management comes from interventions that prevent the need for hospitalization.

As with the frequency of inpatient services, reported hospital charges for individual RSV-related hospitalizations vary widely, from $2,025 to $166,375 in one institution alone.[84] Other reported estimates of hospital charges are $10,236,[85] $27,101,[84] $68,067,[86] and $77,666.[83] These charges cover hospital resource utilization—ie, personnel, intensive care, ventilation, oxygen, specialized respiratory therapy, medications, and other medical services—for 1 hospital stay. Related physician fees and the expense for subsequent ambulatory and/or institutional care that is required by many infants in the 6 to 12 months immediately before and after the initial RSV hospitalization, and the charges for outpatient services that are dedicated to the treatment of nonhospitalized RSV-infected infants are not included in such calculations. For these reasons, the reported charges for a single hospitalization may substantially underestimate the full economic impact of a single RSV episode.

In addition, the cost of managing subsequent reactive airway disease, one of the suggested but incompletely established sequelae of early RSV infections,[46,87-91] has not been accurately determined or factored into economic analyses. Likewise, most indirect and intangible costs of RSV infection generally have been overlooked or remain undetermined. Although these costs may be substantial for parents and families of infected infants and children, they do not impact directly on provider or insurer budgets and, consequently, are of little interest to them.

Cost of Ambulatory Care

The cost of outpatient care, which may constitute as much as 40% of total direct medical expenditures, has been determined through a retrospective survey-based study conducted among parents or caregivers of infants ≤24 months of age with presumed RSV infection.[92] Of the 43 infants assessed, 42 (97.7%) required respiratory-related ambulatory care from generalists and/or specialists in emergency departments and/or urgent-care facilities. Ten infants who received RSV-IGIV required an average of 6.1 visits, while the remaining 33 infants who did not receive RSV-IGIV required an average of 8.6 visits. The average costs for a primary care physician visit (including urgent care) were $372 and $477 for prophylaxed and nonprophylaxed infants, respectively. Similarly, prophylaxed and nonprophylaxed infants had an average cost of $86 and $242, respectively, for an emergency department visit; $9 and $41, respectively, for a specialist; and $241 and $517, respectively, for medications. Total average ambulatory costs were $707 for prophylaxed infants and $1,277 for nonprophylaxed infants. Resource utilization and costs were also stratified by such patient characteristics as comorbidities and gestational age.

Estimates of similar expenses were also reported in a study to establish the expected cost of outpatient care for premature infants with mild-to-severe infections.[93] Based on survey responses from highly experienced physicians, the total expected outpatient costs for prophylaxed and nonprophylaxed infants were $69 and $643, respectively.

Table 2: Relative Cost-Effectiveness of Medical Interventions

Medical Intervention	Cost per Life Year Saved
Autologous blood donation	$235,000
Pneumococcal vaccination	$80,000
Pulmonary artery catheterization	$77,404
RSV-IGIV prophylaxis	$24,305
Breast cancer screening	$18,955
Hydrochlorothiazide for hypertension	$16,400
β-blocker for myocardial infarction	$5,900

Indirect Costs

Direct nonmedical and indirect costs were also included in the retrospective survey-based study.[92] Higher costs for transportation and lost work were incurred by parents and/or caregivers of nonprophylaxed, compared to prophylaxed, infants. The average transportation expense for parents of infants who received RSV-IGIV prophylaxis was $178, compared to $224 for parents of infants who did not. Parents of prophylaxed infants lost an average of $168 in wages, whereas parents of nonprophylaxed infants lost $758. Average baby-sitter costs for both groups of parents were similar ($93 each). Combined, these costs added up to $439 for caregivers and/or parents of prophylaxed infants, and $1,075 for caregivers and/or parents of nonprophylaxed infants.

Cost and Benefit Studies of RSV Immune Globulin and Monoclonal Antibody

Data from a randomized multicenter clinical trial to assess the safety and efficacy of RSV immune globulin in high-risk infants and young children were used in a decision algorithm model for cost-effectiveness expressed as cost per life year saved.[52] The net average cost for immunoprophylaxis was $4,460 for a survival benefit of 0.1835 years of life, resulting in a cost of $24,305 per life year saved. If disease mortality was affected only through a reduction in hospitalization rates, then the survival benefit was 0.1448 years of life, resulting in a cost of $30,805 per life year saved. Model results were robust across reasonable variations in the study parameters that were selected for sensitivity analysis. The cost-effectiveness ratios compared favorably with those of other standard medical interventions (Table 2).

The economics of RSV-IGIV prophylaxis of preterm, very low birth-weight infants and infants with bronchopulmonary dysplasia were assessed from a payer's perspective using outcome data from a randomized trial[22] and cost data from a tertiary-care center.[94] The frequencies of RSV-related hospitalization were 12% for preterm infants without bronchopulmonary dysplasia, 17% for preterm infants with mild bronchopulmonary dysplasia, and 28% for preterm infants with moderate-to-severe bronchopulmonary dysplasia. Five doses of RSV-IGIV were estimated to cost $3,280 to $8,800, based on infant weight (1.2 kg to 10.0 kg) at the time of the initial dose. Estimated net costs for prophylaxis ranged from $5,415 for an infant without bronchopulmonary dysplasia weighing 6 kg, to $1,689 for an infant with bronchopulmonary dysplasia, aged <3 months. The average duration of stay for hospitalized infants was 5 days at a daily cost of $971, for a total of $4,855. Although the hospitalization rate of immunoglobulin recipients was reduced by 41% in the clinical trial, the cost of RSV-IGIV prophylaxis exceeded the benefit of hospitalizations prevented by several thousand dollars. The incremental costs associated with RSV-IGIV were lower for infants with bronchopulmonary dysplasia and for infants <3 months of age.

Based on data from 3 randomized controlled trials, a number-needed-to-treat analysis was performed to estimate how many infants must be prophylaxed with RSV-IGIV to avoid 1 hospital admission for RSV infection.[95] Results were reported as a threshold number that balanced costs related to prophylaxis with dollar benefits related to avoided hospitalizations. Although the range of threshold values was broad (63 for premature infants without chronic lung disease to 12 for those with bronchopulmonary dysplasia), the average was 16, meaning that 16 infants must be prophylaxed with RSV-IGIV in order to avoid 1 hospital admission. For cost parity in this study, the expense to prophylax 16 infants must equal the expense of 1 hospitalization.

A cost-benefit analysis of RSV-IGIV in high-risk infants showed that RSV-IGIV is cost-effective for infants with bronchopulmonary dysplasia.[84] The objective of the study was to quantify the costs of RSV-related hospitalization of high-risk infants, and to project the expected cost of providing RSV immunoprophylaxis. In summary, RSV-IGIV was found to be cost-effective when limited to the prophylaxis of high-risk infants with active bronchopulmonary dysplasia who are at increased risk of mortality from RSV lower respiratory tract infection.

In another cost-effectiveness and number-needed-to-treat analysis, 3 strategies—RSV-IGIV, palivizumab, and no prophylaxis—were compared from the societal perspective.[96] Based on an assumed mortality rate of 1.2% among hospitalized premature infants, palivizumab was more effective and less costly than RSV-IGIV. Cost-effectiveness varied by subgroup, with palivizumab being most cost-effective for infants ≤32 weeks' gestational age who had a neonatal intensive care oxygen requirement of ≤28 days. For this group, the cost per hospitalization avoided was $12,000; cost-effectiveness was expressed as $33,000 per life year saved; and the number-needed-to-treat to avoid 1 hospital visit was 7.4 infants. For other subgroups, the cost per hospitalization avoided ranged from $39,000 to $420,000; cost-effectiveness ranged from $110,000 to $1,200,000 per life year saved; and the number-needed-to-treat to avoid 1 hospital visit ranged from 15 to 152 infants.

A payer-perspective expected-charge study was conducted with a decision tree populated with clinical trial data and information abstracted from published reports.[93] For infants at risk for RSV infection, the model depicted 2 alternatives (prophylaxis with palivizumab or no prophylaxis), revealed the clinical consequences of each alternative, and exposed clinical pathways and necessary resources for infants receiving either alternative. The model also estimated the anticipated charges of each alternative. Outcomes data came predominantly from the IMpact clinical trial, in which palivizumab was evaluated for safety and efficacy in preventing hospitalizations caused by RSV infection in preterm infants, including those with bronchopulmonary dysplasia.[23] Frequency data for hospitalizations were abstracted from several clinical studies of RSV prophylaxis to establish a weighted combined hospitalization rate of 12.3% for nonprophylaxed infants, compared with 4.8% for infants prophylaxed with palivizumab.[21,22] These rates were then compared to others that had been previously reported, and modeled against hospital charges; these ranged from $10,236 to $166,375, respectively.[84,85] The expected RSV-related expenses per prophylaxed infant were $4,575 to $31,789, whereas similar expenses for nonprophylaxed infants were $1,116 to $70,896. Therefore, incremental charges of $3,459 (lowest) to savings of $39,107 (highest) can be expected with the widespread clinical use of palivizumab. Eliminating the upper and lower quartiles, the range of expected charges to payers was $5,272 to $15,456 for the palivizumab arm, and $2,904 to $29,017 for the no-prophylaxis arm. When the analysis was refreshed with data from a prospective, single-arm, open-label trial (3.7% hospitalization rate for prophylaxed infants)[61] and a retrospective chart review (2.3% hospitalization rate for prophylaxed infants),[62] expected expenditures ranged from $4,531 to $28,954, respectively, and from $4,391 to $19,742 for prophylaxed infants, based on the full range of hospital charges used in the original assessment.

RSV Infection and Reactive Airway Disease

The link between RSV bronchiolitis in infancy and reactive airway disease later in life has long been suspected.[97] On the physiologic level, a disruption of the neural mechanisms that control respiratory smooth muscle may be one possible explanation for the connection between RSV infection and airway hyperreactivity.[98,99] Immunologic mechanisms may also contribute. Interleukin-11 (IL-11) from RSV-stimulated respiratory epithelial cells may provoke hyperreactivity and bronchospasm directly or indirectly through enhanced production of peptides that cause smooth muscle to contract.[100] Other cytokines have also been implicated in the process.[101]

On the clinical level, wheezing and increased airway reactivity, as well as abnormal pulmonary function and lower arterial oxygen tension, were reported years after severe RSV lower respiratory tract infection in infancy. Retrospective studies compared infants with previous hospitalizations for RSV lower respiratory tract infections, to normal controls who were appropriately matched.[77,90,102] Excessive bronchial reactivity was 3.5 times more common among RSV patients, compared to the controls (25% vs 7%), and wheezing occurred 3 times to 14 times more often. Other studies conducted prospectively also examined the link between severe RSV bronchiolitis in infancy and respiratory disease during childhood.[103-108] They reported that asthma, wheezing, and/or recurrent lower respiratory tract ailments developed in 23% to 92% of infants and children previously afflicted with RSV-related bronchiolitis, and that reactive airway disease occurred in 23% to 67% of such patients.

Based on these findings, a connection between severe RSV lower respiratory tract infection early in life and subsequent reactive pulmonary disease seems likely. Such a connection has economic implications that could impact the cost and benefit of health-care products and services that alter the incidence and course of RSV infection in infants and children. For example, an estimated 14.6 million Americans have asthma, and consume approximately $9.2 billion in direct health-care resources each year.[109] Of the total expense, 54.4% comes from hospitalization, 15.9% from prescribed medications, 12% from office visits, 11% from hospital outpatient care, and 6.8% from emergency department service. Although the average annual cost per patient is $628.80, this figure is deceiving because 20% of patients account for 80% of the direct medical expenditures, amounting to $2,584 per patient per year. Obviously, any health-care intervention that could reduce the incidence of asthma would also reduce the total economic burden of the illness. The savings would accrue as an economic benefit of the intervention, and would help to defray its cost in use.

Analyses to determine the potential economic benefit derived from a reduction in reactive airway disease would require the following data: 1) a definitive connection between early RSV infection and subsequent airway hyperreactivity; 2) an estimate of the annual incidence of RSV-related hyperreactivity and its natural history; 3) an estimate of the potential reduction in the annual incidence through RSV prophylaxis; 4) per-child annual expense for reactive airway disease; 5) total potential annual savings resulting from any prophylaxis-related reduction; 6) total potential overall savings; and 7) the dollar value of the savings discounted at a reasonable rate per year. Projections of the positive impact of RSV prophylaxis on the burden of illness of reactive airway disease during childhood could shed new light on the costs and benefits of RSV-IGIV and palivizumab. Considering the projected impact, could RSV-IGIV and palivizumab therapy universally lead to overall cost savings when all at-risk populations are protected? If not, where is the threshold for cost parity?

Conclusion

Health economic analyses of RSV infection, management of infected infants, and the passive immunity achieved with palivizumab depend on many factors. Because information on the potential long-term sequelae of early RSV infections is still forthcoming, data on hospitalization rates and initial charges associated with acute RSV-related lower respiratory infection, in large part, determine the current burden of illness. Hospitalization rates were substantially lower in clinical trials than in observational studies, and initial hospital charges constituted only a portion of the total expenses incurred by infected infants. Secondary and, possibly even tertiary, hospital stays would substantially increase the expense of treating infections, and would strengthen the rationale for interventions that protect infants against RSV, ultimately reducing the need for institutional care.

Obviously, costs related to prophylaxis and the treatment of infections are dependent on the duration of the study and the resources that are consumed during the full period of care. If neonatal RSV infection is truly linked to reactive airway disease, then resource consumption for affected individuals would be prolonged, as would the related expense. Finally, the size (approximately 325,000 infants per season in the United States alone) and demographics of at-risk populations dramatically influence calculations. If all at-risk infants are prophylaxed, costs and benefits would be maximized; if palivizumab is given only to infants with the greatest risk, prophylactic costs and overall benefits would be minimized.

Discussion

In the past, clinical decisions were made on the basis of medical need, as well as the safety and efficacy of potentially applied resources. Today, in view of financial constraints that exist in many health-care environments, choices should also be based on sound economic information about alternative options for patient care in order to achieve the greatest outcomes at least resource cost. Consequently, providers, payers, and patients, along with health-related industries and government agencies, are taking a more active interest and assuming expanded roles in health economics research. Their aims are to measure the clinical and economic costs and benefits that are associated with a growing array of health-care interventions, and to meet the medical needs of a health-conscious and cost-conscious public with the finest products and services currently available. The challenge has been and continues to be matching available funds to widespread needs that exist on a global level.

Beyond these considerations are the humanistic and ethical concerns that should be a part of any decision regarding patient care. Are all patients in a society equally valued and equally managed within the health-care arena? What level of clinical effectiveness justifies the clinical use of a product or service? Which medical expenses are justifiable, or unjustifiable? Is the rationing of health care acceptable on any level, for any reason? The answers to these questions teeter in the balance of societal and individual needs, the wealth of the society, and the inherent values of its members. By revealing the comparative costs and benefits of health-care interventions through health economics research, we can begin to understand some of the complexities that underlie these questions and contribute to their answers. Moreover, we gain a greater appreciation of ways to expand access to care through greater efficiency and cost-effectiveness.

References

1. Darville T, Yamauchi T: Respiratory syncytial virus. *Pediatr Rev* 1998;19:55-61.

2. Hall CB, McCarthy CA: Respiratory syncytial virus. In: Mandell GL, Bennett JE, Dolin R, eds. *Mandell, Douglas and Bennett's Principles and Practice of Infectious Diseases.* 4th ed. New York, NY, Churchill Livingstone Inc, 1995, pp 1501-1519.

3. Welliver RC, Ogra PL: Respiratory syncytial virus. In: Gorbach SL, Bartlett JG, Blacklow NR, Zorab R, eds. *Infectious Diseases.* 2nd ed. Philadelphia, PA, WB Saunders Company, 1998, pp 2148-2155.

4. Long CE, McBride JT, Hall CB: Sequelae of respiratory syncytial virus infections: A role for intervention studies. *Am J Respir Crit Care Med* 1995;151:1678-1681.

5. Heilman CA: From the National Institute of Allergy and Infectious Diseases and the World Health Organization. Respiratory syncytial and parainfluenza viruses. *J Infect Dis* 1990;161:402-406.

6. Simoes EA: Epidemiology of respiratory syncytial virus infection: a global perspective. *Infect Med* 1999;16(suppl C):21-24.

7. Holberg CJ, Wright AL, Martinez FD, et al: Risk factors for respiratory syncytial virus-associated lower respiratory illnesses in the first year of life. *Am J Epidemiol* 1991;133:1135-1151.

8. Groothuis JR, Gutierrez KM, Laver BA: Respiratory syncytial virus infection in children with bronchopulmonary dysplasia. *Pediatrics* 1988;82:199-203.

9. Hall CB, Powell KR, MacDonald NE, et al: Respiratory syncytial viral infection in children with compromised immune function. *N Engl J Med* 1986;315:77-81.

10. Yüksel B, Greenough A: Birth weight and hospital readmission of infants born prematurely. *Arch Pediatr Adolesc Med* 1994;148:384-388.

11. Cunningham CK, McMillan JA, Gross SJ: Rehospitalization for respiratory illness in infants of less than 32 weeks' gestation. *Pediatrics* 1991;88:527-532.

12. MacDonald NE, Hall CB, Suffin SC, et al: Respiratory syncytial viral infection in infants with congenital heart disease. *N Engl J Med* 1982;307:397-400.

13. Wang EE, Law BJ, Stephens D: Pediatric Investigators Collaborative Network on Infections in Canada (PICNIC) prospective study of risk factors and outcomes in patients hospitalized with respiratory syncytial viral lower respiratory tract infection. *J Pediatr* 1995;126:212-219.

14. Crowe JE Jr, Bui PT, Firestone CY, et al: Live subgroup B respiratory syncytial virus vaccines that are attenuated, genetically stable, and immunogenic in rodents and nonhuman primates. *J Infect Dis* 1996;173:829-839.

15. Dudas RA, Karron RA: Respiratory syncytial virus vaccines. *Clin Microbiol Rev* 1998;11:430-439.

16. Groothuis JR, King SJ, Hogerman DA, et al: Safety and immunogenicity of a purified F protein respiratory syncytial virus (PFP-2) vaccine in seropositive children with bronchopulmonary dysplasia. *J Infect Dis* 1998;177:467-469.

17. Piedra PA, Grace S, Jewell A, et al: Sequential annual administration of purified fusion protein vaccine against respiratory syncytial virus in children with cystic fibrosis. *Pediatr Infect Dis J* 1998;17:217-224.

18. Karron RA, Wright PF, Crowe JE Jr, et al: Evaluation of two live, cold-passaged, temperature-sensitive respiratory syncytial virus vaccines in chimpanzees and in human adults, infants, and children. *J Infect Dis* 1997;176:1428-1436.

19. Pringle CR, Filipiuk AH, Robinson BS, et al: Immunogenicity and pathogenicity of a triple temperature-sensitive modified respiratory syncytial virus in adult volunteers. *Vaccine* 1993;11:473-478.

20. Tristram DA, Welliver RC, Mohar CK, et al: Immunogenicity and safety of respiratory syncytial virus subunit vaccine in seropositive children 18-36 months old. *J Infect Dis* 1993;167:191-195.

21. Groothuis JR, Simoes EA, Levin MJ, et al: Prophylactic administration of respiratory syncytial virus immune globulin to high-risk infants and young children. *N Engl J Med* 1993;329:1524-1530.

22. Reduction of respiratory syncytial virus hospitalization among premature infants and infants with bronchopulmonary dysplasia using respiratory syncytial virus immune globulin prophylaxis. The PREVENT Study Group. *Pediatrics* 1997;99:93-99.

23. Palivizumab, a humanized respiratory syncytial virus monoclonal antibody, reduces hospitalization from respiratory syncy-

tial virus infection in high-risk infants. The IMpact-RSV Study Group. *Pediatrics* 1998;102:531-537.

24. American Academy of Pediatrics Committee on Infectious Diseases: Respiratory Syncytial Virus. In: Peter G, ed. *1997 Red Book: Report of the Committee on Infectious Diseases*. 24th ed. Elk Grove Village, IL, American Academy of Pediatrics,1997, pp 443-447.

25. Culyer AJ: The morality of efficiency in health care—some uncomfortable implications. *Health Econ* 1992;1:7-18.

26. Sonoda S, Gotoh Y, Bann F, et al: Acute lower respiratory infections in hospitalized children over a 6-year period in Tokyo. *Pediatr Int* 1999;41:519-524.

27. Update: respiratory syncytial virus activity—United States, 1998-1999 season. *MMWR Morb Mortal Wkly Rep* 1999;48:1104-1106, 1115.

28. Izurieta HS, Thompson WW, Kramarz P, et al: Influenza and the rates of hospitalization for respiratory disease among infants and young children. *N Engl J Med* 2000;342:232-239.

29. Shay DK, Holman RC, Newman RD, et al: Bronchiolitis-associated hospitalizations among US children, 1980-1996. *JAMA* 1999;282:1440-1446.

30. De Boeck K: Respiratory syncytial virus bronchiolitis: clinical aspects and epidemiology. *Monaldi Arch Chest Dis* 1996;51: 210-213.

31. Kellner JD, Ohlsson A, Gadomski AM, et al: Efficacy of bronchodilator therapy in bronchiolitis. A meta-analysis. *Arch Pediatr Adolesc Med* 1996;150:1166-1172.

32. Sanchez I, De Koster J, Powell RE, et al: Effect of racemic epinephrine and salbutamol on clinical score and pulmonary mechanics in infants with bronchiolitis. *J Pediatr* 1993;122:145-151.

33. Menon K, Sutcliffe T, Klassen TP: A randomized trial comparing the efficacy of epinephrine with salbutamol in the treatment of acute bronchiolitis. *J Pediatr* 1995;126:1004-1007.

34. Hall CB, McBride JT, Walsh EE, et al: Aerosolized ribavirin treatment of infants with respiratory syncytial viral infection: a randomized double-blind study. *N Engl J Med* 1983;308: 1443-1447.

35. Randolph AG, Wang EE: Ribavirin for respiratory syncytial virus lower respiratory tract infection: a systematic overview. *Arch Pediatr Adolesc Med* 1996;150:942-947.

36. Smith DW, Frankel LR, Mathers LH, et al: A controlled trial of aerosolized ribavirin in infants receiving mechanical ventilation for severe respiratory syncytial virus infection. *N Engl J Med* 1991;325:24-29.

37. Meert KL, Sarnaik AP, Gelmini MJ, et al: Aerosolized ribavirin in mechanically ventilated children with respiratory syncytial virus lower respiratory tract disease: a prospective, double-blind, randomized trial. *Crit Care Med* 1994;22:566-572.

38. Krilov LR, Mandel FS, Barone SR, et al: Follow-up of children with respiratory syncytial virus bronchiolitis in 1986 and 1987: potential effect of ribavirin on long term pulmonary function. *Pediatr Infect Dis J* 1997;16:273-276.

39. Ventura F, Cheseaux JJ, Cotting J, et al: Is the use of ribavirin aerosols in respiratory syncytial virus infections justified? Clinical and economic evaluation. *Arch Pediatr* 1998;5:123-131.

40. Ohmit SE, Moler FW, Monto AS, et al: Ribavirin utilization and clinical effectiveness in children hospitalized with respiratory syncytial virus infection. *J Clin Epidemiol* 1996;49:963-967.

41. Moler FW, Steinhart CM, Ohmit SE, et al: Effectiveness of ribavirin in otherwise well infants with respiratory syncytial virus-associated respiratory failure. *J Pediatr* 1996;128:422-428.

42. Law BJ, Wang EE, MacDonald N, et al: Does ribavirin impact on the hospital course of children with respiratory syncytial virus (RSV) infection? An analysis using the Pediatric Investigators Collaborative Network on Infections in Canada (PICNIC) RSV database. *Pediatrics* 1997;99:E7.

43. De Boeck K, Van der AN, Van Lierde S, et al: Respiratory syncytial virus bronchiolitis: a double-blind dexamethasone efficacy study. *J Pediatr* 1997;131:919-921.

44. Bulow SM, Nir M, Levin E, et al: Prednisolone treatment of respiratory syncytial virus infection: a randomized controlled trial of 147 infants. *Pediatrics* 1999;104:e77.

45. Roosevelt G, Sheehan K, Grupp-Phelan J, et al: Dexamethasone in bronchiolitis: a randomised controlled trial. *Lancet* 1996;348:292-295.

46. Abman SH, Ogle JW, Butler-Simon N, et al: Role of respiratory syncytial virus in early hospitalizations for respiratory dis-

tress of young infants with cystic fibrosis. *J Pediatr* 1988;113:826-830.

47. Green M, Brayer AF, Schenkman KA, et al: Duration of hospitalization in previously well infants with respiratory syncytial virus infection. *Pediatr Infect Dis J* 1989;8:601-605.

48. AARC (American Association for Respiratory Care) clinical practice guideline. Oxygen therapy in the acute care hospital. *Respir Care* 1991;36:1410-1413.

49. Gandy, A: Pediatric Database (PEDBASE); accessed June 1, 2000. Web address: *www.icondata.com/health/pedbase/pedlynx.htm.*

50. Slutsky AS: Mechanical ventilation. American College of Chest Physicians' Consensus Conference. *Chest* 1993;104:1833-1859.

51. Fraser J, Henrichsen T, Mok Q, et al: Prolonged mechanical ventilation as a consequence of acute illness. *Arch Dis Child* 1998;78:253-256.

52. Hay JW, Ernst RL, Meissner HC: Respiratory syncytial virus immune globulin: a cost effectiveness analysis. *Am J Man Care* 1996;2:851-861.

53. Hall CB, Powell KR, Schnabel KC, et al: Risk of secondary bacterial infection in infants hospitalized with respiratory syncytial viral infection. *J Pediatr* 1988;113:266-271.

54. Collins PL, McIntosh K, Chanock M: Respiratory syncytial virus. In: Fields BN, Knipe DM, Howley PM, eds. *Fields Virology.* 3rd ed. New York, NY, Lippencott-Raven, 1996, pp 1212-1351.

55. Arnold SR, Wang EE, Law BJ, et al: Variable morbidity of respiratory syncytial virus infection in patients with underlying lung disease: a review of the PICNIC RSV database. *Pediatr Infect Dis J* 1999;18:866-869.

56. Hiatt PW, Grace SC, Kozinetz CA, et al: Effects of viral lower respiratory tract infection on lung function in infants with cystic fibrosis. *Pediatrics* 1999;103:619-626.

57. Simoes EA: Respiratory syncytial virus infection. *Lancet* 1999;354:847-852.

58. La Via WV, Grant SW, Stutman HR, et al: Clinical profile of pediatric patients hospitalized with respiratory syncytial virus infection. *Clin Pediatr (Phila)* 1993;32:450-454.

59. Behrendt CE, Decker MD, Burch DJ, et al: International variation in the management of infants hospitalized with respiratory syncytial virus. *Eur J Pediatr* 1998;157:215-220.

60. Simoes EA, Groothuis JR, Tristram DA, et al: Respiratory syncytial virus-enriched globulin for the prevention of acute otitis media in high risk children . *J Pediatr* 1996;129:214-219.

61. Law B, Andre P, Baarsma R, et al: Palivizumab (Synagis™) expanded access study in 1998-99—Northern hemisphere. Presented at the Second World Congress of Pediatric Infectious Diseases, Manila, Philippines, 1999. Abstract P25.

62. Cohen A, Hirsch RL, Sorrentino M, et al: First year experience using Synagis™ palivizumab humanized monoclonal antibody for protection from RSV lower respiratory tract infection. Presented at the Second World Congress of Pediatric Infectious Diseases, Manila, Philippines, 1999. Abstract A16.

63. Rodriguez WJ, Arrobio J, Fink R, et al: Prospective follow-up and pulmonary functions from a placebo-controlled randomized trial of ribavirin therapy in respiratory syncytial virus bronchiolitis. *Arch Pediatr Adolesc Med* 1999;153:469-474.

64. Reassessment of the indications for ribavirin therapy in respiratory syncytial virus infections. American Academy of Pediatrics Committee on Infectious Diseases. *Pediatrics* 1996;97:137-140.

65. Edell D, Bruce E, Hale K, et al: Reduced long-term respiratory morbidity after treatment of respiratory syncytial virus bronchiolitis with ribavirin in previously healthy infants: a preliminary report. *Pediatr Pulmonol* 1998;25:154-158.

66. Long CE, Voter KZ, Barker WH, et al: Long-term follow-up of children hospitalized with respiratory syncytial virus lower respiratory tract infection and randomly treated with ribavirin or placebo. *Pediatr Infect Dis J* 1997;16:1023-1028.

67. Fergie JE: Effects of ribavirin therapy on RSV infections in high-risk infants and young children 2 years after hospitalization. In: Hiatt PW, ed. *RSV and Asthma: Is There a Link?* New York, NY, American Thoracic Society, 1998, pp 43-45.

68. Gilchrist S, Török TJ, Gary HE, et al: National surveillance for respiratory syncytial virus, United States, 1985-1990. *J Infect Dis* 1994;170:986-990.

69. Kim PE, Musher DM, Glezen WP, et al: Association of invasive pneumococcal disease with season, atmospheric conditions,

air pollution, and the isolation of respiratory viruses. *Clin Infect Dis* 1996;22:100-106.

70. Brandenburg AH, Jeannet PY, Steensel-Moll HA, et al: Local variability in respiratory syncytial virus disease severity. *Arch Dis Child* 1997;77:410-414.

71. Walsh EE, McConnochie KM, Long CE, et al: Severity of respiratory syncytial virus infection is related to virus strain. *J Infect Dis* 1997;175:814-820.

72. Hall CB, Walsh EE, Schnabel KC, et al: Occurrence of groups A and B of respiratory syncytial virus over 15 years: associated epidemiologic and clinical characteristics in hospitalized and ambulatory children. *J Infect Dis* 1990;162:1283-1290.

73. McConnochie KM, Hall CB, Walsh EE, et al: Variation in severity of respiratory syncytial virus infections with subtype. *J Pediatr* 1990;117:52-62.

74. Lehr MV, Simoes EA: A weapon against RSV for children at risk. *Contemp Pediatr* 1998;15:78-90.

75. Wang EE, Law BJ, Boucher FD, et al: Pediatric Investigators Collaborative Network on Infections in Canada (PICNIC) study of admission and management variation in patients hospitalized with respiratory syncytial viral lower respiratory tract infection. *J Pediatr* 1996;129:390-395.

76. Schwartz R: Respiratory syncytial virus in infants and children. *Nurse Pract* 1995;20:24-29.

77. Dezateux C, Fletcher ME, Dundas I, et al: Infant respiratory function after RSV-proven bronchiolitis. *Am J Respir Crit Care Med* 1997;155:1349-1355.

78. Sandritter TL, Kraus DM: Respiratory syncytial virus-immunoglobulin intravenous (RSV-IGIV) for respiratory syncytial viral infections: part I. *J Pediatr Health Care* 1997;11:284-291.

79. Emond A, Evans JA, Howat P: The continuing morbidity and use of health services by preterm infants after discharge from hospital. *Ambulatory Child Health* 1997;3:121-129.

80. Wright AL, Taussig LM, Ray CG, et al: The Tucson Children's Respiratory Study. II. Lower respiratory tract illness in the first year of life. *Am J Epidemiol* 1989;129:1232-1246.

81. Donati D, Cellesi C, Rossolini A, et al: Serological diagnosis of respiratory viral infections. A five-year study of hospitalized patients. *New Microbiol* 1998;21:365-374.

82. Yun BY, Kim MR, Park JY, et al: Viral etiology and epidemiology of acute lower respiratory tract infections in Korean children. *Pediatr Infect Dis J* 1995;14:1054-1059.

83. Langley JM, Wang EE, Law BJ, et al: Economic evaluation of respiratory syncytial virus infection in Canadian children: a Pediatric Investigators Collaborative Network on Infections in Canada (PICNIC) study. *J Pediatr* 1997;131:113-117.

84 Oelberg D, Reininger M, Van Eeckhout J: A cost-benefit analysis of respiratory syncytial virus hyperimmune globulin (RSV-IVIG) in high-risk infants. *Neonatal Intensive Care*. 1998:29-33.

85. Grier CE, Howe BJ: Economic impact of pneumonia due to respiratory syncytial virus (RSV) infection. Presented at the ICAAC 35th Annual Meeting, San Francisco, CA, 1995. Abstract N9.

86. Meissner HC: Economic impact of viral respiratory disease in children. *J Pediatr* 1994;124:S17-S21.

87. Gurwitz D, Mindorff C, Levison H: Increased incidence of bronchial reactivity in children with a history of bronchiolitis. *J Pediatr* 1981;98:551-555.

88. Kattan M, Keens TG, Lapierre JG, et al: Pulmonary function abnormalities in symptom-free children after bronchiolitis. *Pediatrics* 1977;59:683-688.

89. Martinez FD, Wright AL, Taussig LM, et al: Asthma and wheezing in the first six years of life. *N Engl J Med* 1995;332:133-138.

90. Pullan CR, Hey EN: Wheezing, asthma, and pulmonary dysfunction 10 years after infection with respiratory syncytial virus in infancy. *BMJ* 1982;284:1665-1669.

91. Welliver RC: RSV and chronic asthma. *Lancet*.1995;346:789-790.

92. Kaplan-Machlis B, Beane JS: Health care resource utilization and costs of RSV-related hospitalizations. *Neonatal Intensive Care*. 2000;13:17-25.

93. Marchetti A, Lau H, Magar R, et al: Impact of palivizumab on expected costs of respiratory syncytial virus infection in preterm infants: potential for savings. *Clin Ther* 1999;21:752-766.

94. O'Shea TM, Sevick MA, Givner LB: Costs and benefits of respiratory syncytial virus immunoglobulin to prevent hospitalization for lower respiratory tract illness in very low birth weight infants. *Pediatr Infect Dis J* 1998;17:587-593.

95.   Robbins JM, Tilford JM, Jacobs RF, et al: A number-needed-to-treat analysis of the use of respiratory syncytial virus immune globulin to prevent hospitalization. *Arch Pediatr Adolesc Med* 1998;152:358-366.

96.   Joffe S, Escobar GJ, Black SB, et al: Rehospitalization for respiratory syncytial virus among premature infants. *Pediatrics* 1999;104:894-899.

97.   Simoes EA: Respiratory syncytial virus and subsequent lower respiratory tract infections in developing countries. A new twist to an old virus. *J Pediatr* 1999;135:657-661.

98.   Folkerts G, Busse WW, Nijkamp FP, et al: Virus-induced airway hyperresponsiveness and asthma. *Am J Respir Crit Care Med* 1998;157:1708-1720.

99.   Larsen GL: RSV Infection and airway neural control in animal models. In: Hiatt PW, ed. *RSV and Asthma: Is There a Link?* New York, American Thoracic Society, 1998, pp 17-20.

100. Einarsson O, Geba GP, Zhu Z, et al: Interleukin-11: stimulation in vivo and in vitro by respiratory viruses and induction of airways hyperresponsiveness. *J Clin Invest* 1996;97:915-924.

101. Lemanske RF: Immunologic mechanisms in RSV-related allergy and asthma. In: Hiatt PW, ed. *RSV and Asthma: Is There a Link?* New York, American Thoracic Society, 1998, pp 11-16.

102. Sims DG, Downham MA, Gardner PS, et al: Study of 8-year-old children with a history of respiratory syncytial virus bronchiolitis in infancy. *BMJ* 1978;1:11-14.

103. Hall CB, Hall WJ, Gala CL, et al: Long-term prospective study in children after respiratory syncytial virus infection. *J Pediatr* 1984;105:358-364.

104. Henry RL, Hodges IG, Milner AD, et al: Respiratory problems 2 years after acute bronchiolitis in infancy. *Arch Dis Child* 1983;58:713-716.

105. Stokes GM, Milner AD, Hodges IG, et al: Lung function abnormalities after acute bronchiolitis. *J Pediatr* 1981;98:871-874.

106. Sly PD, Hibbert ME: Childhood asthma following hospitalization with acute viral bronchiolitis in infancy. *Pediatr Pulmonol* 1989;7:153-158.

107. Webb MS, Henry RL, Milner AD, et al: Continuing respiratory problems three and a half years after acute viral bronchiolitis. *Arch Dis Child* 1985;60:1064-1067.

108. Rooney JC, Williams HE: The relationship between proved viral bronchiolitis and subsequent wheezing. *J Pediatr* 1971;79:744-747.

109. Smith DH, Malone DC, Lawson KA, et al: A national estimate of the economic costs of asthma. *Am J Respir Crit Care Med* 1997;156:787-793.

Index

A

lymphocytic hyperresponsiveness 106

lymphocytic peribronchiolar infiltration 73, 184

lymphoproliferative activity 106

M

macrophage inflammatory proteins (MIPs) 95, 96, 98-100, 104, 105, 109

macrophages 96, 100, 109
  alveolar 109

malaise 81

malnutrition 49

marrow engraftment 54

mast cells 109

measles vaccine 163

measles virus 142, 153, 180

mechanical ventilation 49, 51, 52, 82, 137, 139, 142, 143, 146, 160, 161, 167, 211-214, 218, 222

MedImmune, Inc. 164, 170, 190

Merck Institute for Therapeutic Research 13

MHC-1 antigens 96

microneutralizing antibody titers 27, 28, 59

monoclonal antibody (MAb) 18, 19, 27, 95, 126, 128, 164-166, 176, 190

monocyte chemotactic proteins (MCPs) 96, 98, 99, 105

monocytes 98

Morris CCA report 10

Morris, JA 10

mucosal biopsies 97

mumps vaccine 163

myasthenia gravis 143

Mycoplasma pneumoniae 13

myeloperoxidase 100

myocardial infarction 224

N

nasal congestion 76, 78, 80

nasal epithelial biopsy 99

nasal lavage specimens 25

nasal mucosa 46, 72

nasal secretions 10, 46, 100, 102, 108, 123, 159

nasal swabs 123

nasal wash 123, 127, 210, 217

nasopharyngeal aspirates 210

nasopharyngeal cells 123, 126

NOTES